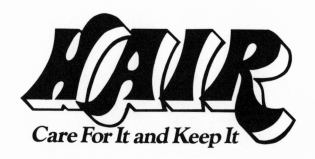

Care For It and Keep It

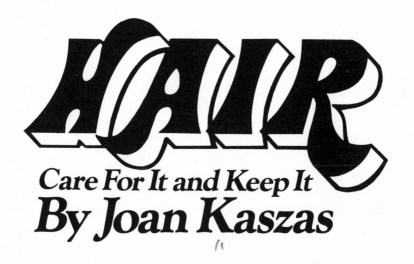

Care For It and Keep It
By Joan Kaszas

**Nash Publishing
Los Angeles**

Library of Congress Catalog Card Number: 72-95245
Standard Book Number: 8402-1275-5

Published simultaneously in the United States and Canada
by Nash Publishing Corporation, 9255 Sunset Boulevard,
Los Angeles, California 90069.

Printed in the United States of America.

First Printing.

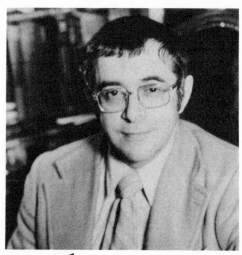

Foreword

That slender sliver that graces one's scalp has from the beginning of time served as a protective matter, a figure of enticement (i.e., Texas Guinan, red-haired; Marilyn Monroe, blonde; Cleopatra, black), and even a symbol of strength as biblically related by Samson whom Delilah successfully sheared of his powers by clipping his locks.

Hair, hence, represents virility, strength, beauty, intrigue. It also serves as a major physical evaluation of good health. Strong, shiny, vibrant hair designates good health—as opposed to dry, sparse, weak strands noted in poorly controlled diabetics and in those suffering from malnutrition and debilitating diseases. It is a small wonder that more has not been said or written about hair—its keep, its care, its cosmetic and physical importance.

Miss Kaszas has deeply and thoroughly researched the problems attendant on hair, as well as hair's scientific and pathological relationships. Throughout the entire text detailed evidence of corrective measures have been put forth. The subject of nutrition has been courageously covered as a part of the overall care of hair. It should be noted that the relationship of nutrition and hair is becoming more and more evident in both lay and scientific literature.

The various techniques—such as chemical, mechanical, et cetera—have been selectively updated. Amazingly, Miss Kaszas has discovered so much to relate from so little but so important a sliver of protein called hair. The entire book has intrigue and, indeed, alleviates the lack of knowledge which most of us have about hair.

This book directs attention to improving our hair and emphasizes the fact that we and our hair are one. The entire structure must be holistically approached.

Hair offers a myriad of valuable items of information together with helpful advice. It pays homage to that sliver of protein, hair, and shows how important it really is to all of us.

HAROLD ROSENBERG, M.D.
President of the International
Academy of Preventive Medicine

Contents

Introduction

I first met Joan Kaszas several years ago while visiting a friend in New York. Joan, who lived across the hall, stopped in for a cup of coffee, and I must say I *did* notice her hair, but for all the wrong reasons—it was dull and lifeless with split ends and a gummy quality.

For this reason you can imagine my surprise when just a few months later, the time of our second meeting, Joan's hair was utterly transformed—shining, full of highlights, healthy, bouncy, thick and lovely. I was astounded.

As a model I was naturally interested in all aspects of grooming, clothes, make-up and hair. My work required being up on all the latest developments and fashions; anything new never failed to attract my attention. So of course I had to find out what Joan had done to bring about so miraculous a change—perhaps she had some secrets I'd never heard of?

Taking Joan aside, I asked her pointblank what she'd been doing to herself. Joan replied it would take some time to go into, but we could get together over lunch and she'd tell all.

That's exactly what she did do. I learned that Joan, realizing her own dire straits, had decided to make a thorough study of hair, its care and grooming. In the process, her research had taken her all over the world, to distant places in Europe, the Far East and Africa, where she not only talked to all kinds of official "establishment" people like hairdressers, physicians, pharmacists, chemists, cosmeticians, etc., but also to such esoteric sources as African witch doctors and Hawaiian kahunas. Listening to Joan's adventures is a colorful experience that should someday become a book in itself.

I confessed to Joan that despite the fact that I'd done numerous commercials and acting parts, I was still plagued with problem hair that needed special attention—it was thin, fine, stringy, lacking in body, hard to hold in a set, with ends that tended to split, and it grew slowly. The outline of my problems didn't deter Joan. "Any hair can be improved," she declared.

Joan did indeed have many new things to offer me on hair care that I'd never heard before, all of which—and more—appear in this book.

I decided to apply Joan's new hints to my own hair, with excellent results. Therefore, I can thoroughly recommend this book to any woman interested in improving her appearance—and needless to say I endorse Joan Kaszas's methods wholeheartedly.

—Jeanne Rejaunier

1.
Hair Problems
Why and How They Occur

Experts agree unanimously that the majority of hair and scalp ills are self-inflicted. In a fanatical drive to improve on the work of Mother Nature, most of us tend to overreact to our hair problems. Instead of making improvements, our efforts often wind up as unflattering evidence of hair abuse.

There are conditions, however, under which hair and scalp are punished without any self-help. The abundance of dirt, soot, and general pollution in the air is more detrimental to hair and scalp than ever before. Aggravated by the anxieties and perspiration of rush-hour frustrations, the situation worsens. Hair problems caused by chemicals, soot, and fumes will hopefully be alleviated by government legislation and controls; but until such time as these changes are actually activated and enforced, some amount of hair woes will continue to beset us all, particularly city dwellers. The ability of many inhabitants of rural areas to cultivate lifelong crops of hardy hair may in part be attributed to less nerve-wracking tensions. With city dwellers the pressures of cosmopolitan living sometimes show up in the form of ulcers, other times in hair loss. Hair, it would appear, mirrors not only where you live, it mirrors how you live.

Beware. Mother Nature's fickle streak can make nature work against you as well as for you. Long afternoons in the cold outdoors minus the protection of a hat or scarf give wintry winds their opportunity to play havoc, to tangle hair, and to rob it of its natural oils. A season of too much summer sun and salt air are apt to create faded, parched, strawlike hair. Without taking adequate protective steps, summer sun can bake away both luster and color from your hair.

Although excessive sun takes its toll, the sun in proper amounts may be helpful. Increased temperatures and the sun's natural rays of ozone may well promote the growth of hair— provided the sun is taken in small doses. Seaweed and salt water both can be excellent scalp conditioners, if a protective cream is applied to the hair strands first as a safety measure.

There is direct evidence that climate and location affect hair growth. Sun rays not only stimulate plant growth, hair, too, receives benefits. Scientific studies indicate that in hot areas of the world the rate of hair growth increases. Needless to say, in cold-weather areas, the rate of growth is reduced. In the United States, where clothing and temperature can be controlled, a change in weather does not produce any radical change in hair growth. But for anyone moving his home from the North Pole to an equatorial zone, a dramatic difference in hirsuteness would be visible.

Astrological Influences?

You may not be able to move either heaven or earth, but the sun, stars, and moon do play their part—so say astrologers. Some avid astrology buffs claim hair is an antenna to the moon—that it picks up moon vibrations. As a result, one should never cut hair when the moon is waxing (getting full), since it is then that hair is supposedly in its most active state, sending and receiving vibrations. While the moon is on the wane is the time to have your hair cut, as then hair begins to relax, and is more ready to accept quietly the tortures of the scissors. According to astrology, haircuts are reputed to be most successful when the moon is positioned in a mutable or earthy astrological sign. Faster hair growth can be expected when the hair has been cut while the sun and moon are in opposition to one another; slowest hair growth is said to result when the moon is in the sign of Gemini or Leo, in the third or fourth quarters, with Saturn adversely situated. Permanent waves, straightening, and hair coloring are guaranteed successful by starry-minded believers if the moon is in Aquarius with Venus well positioned. When Mars is adversely positioned, these same processes are likely to fail.

The next time you scream, "What in heaven's name can I do with my hair?" you might run out and buy an astrological calendar. In the meantime, however, for more down-to-earth information on techniques for hair improvement—read on.

2.
How Your
Hair Grows

Hair growth is no longer a mystery. Hair grows from a hair follicle; therefore it is essential to understand the function of a hair follicle and what it is. A follicle is a shallot-shaped pit embedded in the skin of the scalp. At its deepest point is a cylindrical bulb which contains the matrix. Hair is formed within the matrix. This is the only living portion of hair; the hair pushing out through the follicle and extending beyond is composed of dead keratin, a fibrous protein substance, intermixed with colored cells.

The part of the hair we see and attend to is referred to as the shaft. In reality the shaft grows from deep within the scalp. If the shaft is damaged, the depth of the root is such that when hair is torn, pulled or broken, injury will occur only at a superficial level. There will be no real damage at the actual growing point. Since the hair we see is not alive, it is unlikely that existing shafts can be regenerated or that hair color be changed, unless a chemical process is introduced.

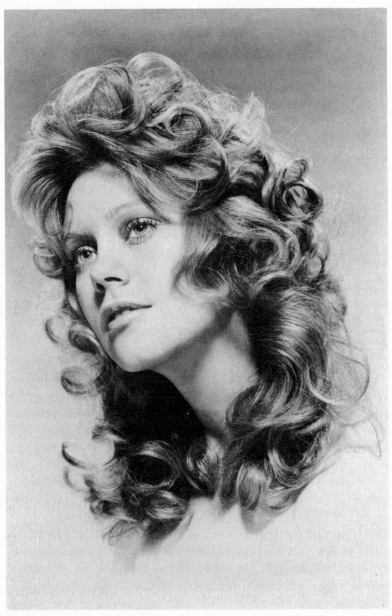

A magnificent head of beautiful hair is not an accident of birth.
Courtesy of Clairol Inc.

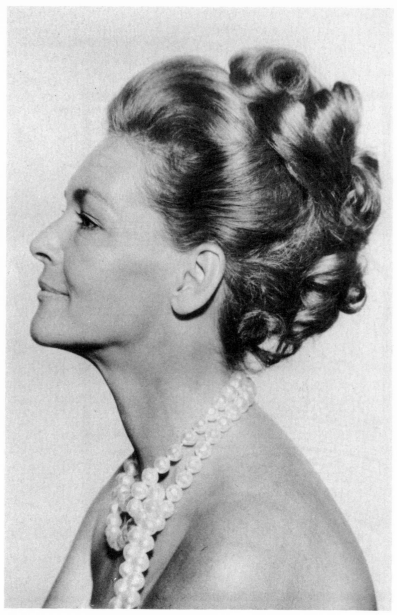

Hair is potentially a great asset. Courtesy of Clairol Inc.

A Hair Follicle—How Your Hair Grows

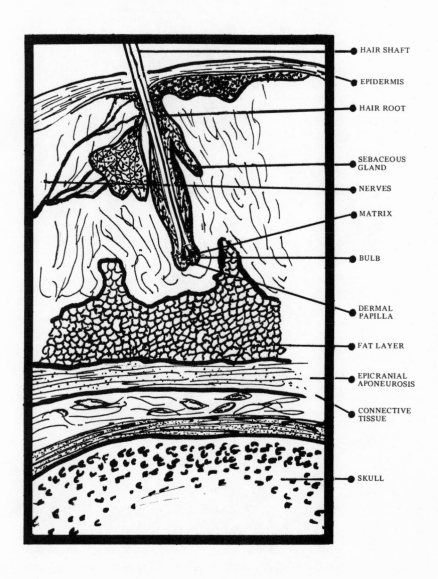

HAIR SHAFT

EPIDERMIS

HAIR ROOT

SEBACEOUS
GLAND

NERVES

MATRIX

BULB

DERMAL
PAPILLA

FAT LAYER

EPICRANIAL
APONEUROSIS

CONNECTIVE
TISSUE

SKULL

Under normal conditions hair grows one-half inch per month or approximately one inch every three months, a total of six inches a year. The rate at which your hair grows goes on regardless of your well- or ill-being. Growth of hair is dependent primarily on the hair follicles receiving adequate nourishment from the body's blood supply. Although health does not control rate of growth, it does affect the growth or no-growth factor, as well as the diameter of the individual hair strands. Hair will be thinner or finer with disease and poor health. With ill health, certain hairs may actually give up growing. Those strands which do grow will do so at a normal pace, but they will look thin, drab, and lifeless.

Hair reflects its own history. Obviously, care and treatment have an influence. Texture and color are inherited traits. Age, too, plays a part. As you mature, so does your hair. Over a span of years your hair color can go from light to dark or dark to light. At any age, hair is, potentially, one of your great assets. At the height of its glory, hair is irresistibly fascinating, magically flexible, mysteriously colorful and absolutely eye-catching. Since hair growth and beauty are dependent on hair follicles receiving nourishment directly from the body's bloodstream, hair constantly mirrors the body's state of health.

3.
Diet, Vitamins, and Your Hair

In order to regain that bright bouncy hair you started out with, pay attention to what is probably the most important single contributor to a healthy head of hair—*proper diet!*

An old adage states, "You are what you eat," which in the simplest of terms means, if you eat quality foods in proper proportions you'll stay in proper shape from the top of your head to the tip of your toes. The preliminary steps in unfolding top-notch beauty and health for you and your hair are (1) rejecting foods which are harmful to the hair and scalp, and (2) switching to those foods which are rich in germinating substances, proteins, minerals and vitamins. These quality foods are absolutely necessary if the body is to produce enzymes and hormones essential for healthy hair growth. The sweet sugary desserts, which you may think are delicious, are normally far from being even slightly nutritious.

A look into the past is necessary to understand what has happened to the food we cram into our hungry mouths. In the days of our great-grandfathers, life was based on "doin' what comes naturally." Grains were not milled, fruits and vegetables were allowed to grow without synthetic fertilizers or chemical additives, animals fed on honest-to-goodness vegetation, fish swam rampant in lakes and streams free of contaminating pollutants. Today it's different. Fish and wildlife are in constant jeopardy due to our polluted waters. Present-day commercial flours are milled virtually to death, stripped of nutritional value. The natural vitamins and minerals found in yesterday's flour—which helped to give great-grandmother's bread its rich delicious taste—have nearly all been lost. Modern-day white breads, white sugar, and white rice are milled, bleached, tortured, and denatured mercilessly, and have almost lost their original wholesomeness. With minor exceptions, the organically grown substances which contributed to the hardy health of our forebearers just do not exist. Backtracking to old ways may offer an answer. Only foods left in their original state retain all of the natural vitamins and minerals which are necessary to promote strong bodies, strong nails, strong teeth, and hardy hair.

Naturally grown, balanced foods, build naturally well-balanced bodies. For example, when too small an amount of organic salt exists in the food we eat, and thus subsequently in the body, vital organs which require these salts make their demands known by stealing salt from less important parts of the body such as hair and nails. It has even been theorized that baldness and lack of hair color may be attributed to a shortage of mineral salts. The best source of mineral salts lies beneath the skin of naturally grown raw foods such as carrots, radishes, celery, cucumbers, etc.

Synthetically fertilized foods lacking their own precious vitamins and minerals, of course, create problems. Surfeited with canned foods and processed meats and cheeses, plus foods and beverages crammed with excesses of white sugar, our diets have become substantially demineralized, denatured, nutritionally deficient, and unbalanced.

If faulty diet can affect hardy organs like teeth and bones, it can and indeed does affect the hair as well. Like teeth and bones, hair is a product of the substances carried within the bloodstream. When impurities are introduced in the bloodstream through demineralization, false fortification, imbalanced foodstuffs, drugs, and gases, repercussions take place. It has been found that whenever the body stores impurities, it attempts to store them in a physically unimportant organ. For this purpose, the scalp is ideal. It has even been theorized that dandruff may be a form of impurity elimination in lieu of adequate normal outlets. Obviously, daily elimination is necessary to rid the body of wastes. One of the culprits responsible for introducing impurities in the bloodstream is the intake of too much food—often of poor nutritional value at that.

The Construction of Hair

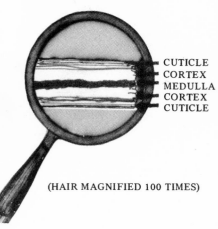

CUTICLE
CORTEX
MEDULLA
CORTEX
CUTICLE

(HAIR MAGNIFIED 100 TIMES)

The Chemistry of Hair

Cuticle: The protective outer layer of hair, composed of flat transparent cells which overlap each other and form a shield for the inner layers. When the cuticle cells lay flat along the shaft, they provide a mirrorlike surface which denotes a healthy structure. Hair damage usually begins with the breakage or wearing away of the cuticle, thereby exposing the soft pulpy cortex.

Medulla: The pithy extreme center of the hair shaft. Often the medulla is absent or formed intermittently through the hair shaft. Its presence is a sign of good health.

Cortex: The soft inner portion which makes up the bulk of hair; where pigment or color is formed. It is also the area where hair gains its elasticity and strength, being composed primarily of proteins.

Here's added health food for thought. In primitive parts of the world, such as the South Seas, Asia, and Africa, where natural foods are still eaten and where modern industrial techniques have not yet struck, hair ills as we know them do not exist. Sans commercial milling and processing, men and women of these so-called backward areas have managed to hang on to their luxurious hair growth.

The Asians manage to promote luxurious hair by adding an age-old ingredient, seaweed, to practically all their dishes. Being brought up from early childhood on a steady diet of fish, soup, salad, and unmilled rice—complemented by the hair-helping minerals and protein of seaweed—makes for the exquisite hair of many Asians.

Nearly every American town has an organic restaurant or health-food store where organic foods may be purchased. If one is not readily handy, careful shopping at the local supermarket and careful reading of labels will head you towards a healthier main course.

Protein

The body—including skin, muscles, internal organs, nails, hair, base of the bones, and even the brain—is largely composed of protein. You are what you eat, remember? Only when protein of excellent quality is supplied can each cell function normally and keep itself in proper repair at all times. Like the muscles within your body, hair which lacks resiliency and elasticity, breaks too easily, or refuses to accept a permanent often will change to healthy hair after just several weeks of improved nutrition.

Eating more protein does not necessarily guarantee more hair, but eating too little protein will definitely produce poor, undernourished hair. In Appalachia, for example, where there is an abundant starch and sugar intake and a definite lack of protein in the diet, hair production is visibly diminished. In recent years it has become more and more evident that a sufficient intake of protein must be included in the diet each and every day in order to maintain a rich and healthy bloodstream.

Animal proteins are considered by nutritionists to be of greater value than the normal vegetable proteins; however, either suffices. Ample sources of daily proteins are available from such easily obtainable foods as fresh milk, cheese, eggs, fish, liver, and kidneys; of course, unprocessed organic protein foods are best.

The popular theory that gelatin supplies a protein of special value for hair has no validity. The protein of gelatin is equivalent to that of chicken, cheese, milk, eggs, or steak. However, if you personally prefer gelatin to a cheese omelet, by all means inform the cook. For those who are interested in their weight as well as their hair, the advantage of gelatin is merely a lower calorie count.

What about quickly liquid lunches? Studies reveal that iced liquids, alcoholic or otherwise, tend to constrict the stomach's blood vessels, as well as the smaller intestines. This result adversely affects blood circulation throughout the body and ultimately interferes with the flow of a healthy blood supply to the scalp and hair follicles, all of which is detrimental to the health and beauty of hair. Drinks prepared at room temperature, slightly warmed or slightly cooled, are less likely to constrict vessels and hinder circulation. It is also important to chew solid foods sufficiently. Doing so helps to eliminate the possibility that alimentary tract disorders may interfere with circulation. The combination of poor chewing habits and consumption of excessive quantities of alcohol, tea, or coffee seriously adds to circulatory problems.

If you must drink, choose distilled liquors such as gin, vodka, or scotch—with diet mixers. Avoid champagne and sweet liqueurs; they are too high in carbohydrates for any hair-improvement diet. Try bits of cheese, unprocessed. Before you wind up an egghead, switch to fertile eggs. A fertile egg is best, but even a supermarket egg is better than none. In any form at all, eggs supply a sizable boost toward meeting the day's nutritional needs. One solitary egg will supply as much protein as an ounce of cooked lean meat. Egg whites being virtually fat-free can be consumed by those watching both weight and health. (Two whole eggs contain a slim 160 calories.)

Egg yolks offer a rich source of iron and vitamin A, both important hair-helpers. When utilized as a main dish, each serving should contain three eggs—or two eggs plus an ounce of cheese, fish, or meat per serving—in order to meet the minimum requirement of three ounces of meat or its equivalent per main dish. A balanced diet is one in which the following general proportions are maintained: 1/4 protein and fat; 1/4 natural sugar and starches; and the remainder vegetables and fruits.

For a delicious and nutritious morning hair-raiser, pop a raw egg into your blender, add milk and a little fresh fruit (no syrup or canned fruit if you know what's good for you); then add a topping of wheat germ. Turn the blender on high, or beat by hand until the drink appears frothy. Without being sickeningly sweet or chemically processed, your homemade shake —undenatured, and chock full of protein—promises to taste as good as it looks, and to impart its delicious health ingredients to the body and hair. An egg shake each morning can give you a head start for a better head of hair.

Fats

A diet which lacks fat intake can also cause nutritional deficiency, affecting both body and hair. Vegetable-oil products, cream, butter, and lard are principal sources of fatty acids which, like proteins, are essential for proper nutrition.

As an example of what infinite care, proper diet, and vigorous daily exercise can produce, think of a beautiful show horse. Good horse sense should tell you that his sensational coat is no mere accident. Forty-five minutes of every day are specially devoted to the grooming, combing, and brushing of a fine show horse. Add to this care, good undenatured feed, vitamin supplements, and healthy doses of fatty cod-liver oil, and the result is an animal with an exquisitely glossy mane and glowing coat, epitomizing all the benefits of proper care and diet.

The hair of man and mouse is not all that different, either. The findings of Dr. George O. Burr, former director of physiological chemistry at the University of Minnesota, exemplify the reverse effects caused by improper diet. Undernourishing diets fed to mice and rats left these poor creatures with dry, thin, scaly, virtually hairless bodies.

Experiments carried out with humans have demonstrated that dry, lifeless hair can be revived and given new luster and gloss when one or two tablespoons of salad oil are added to a daily diet.

Summing it up; you need fats to help burn up protein and to keep your hair and body sleek and strong. The quantity should be nominal. Vegetables generally benefit hair—except for beets, which are high in sugar, and potatoes and lima beans, both high in carbohydrates. Fruits have a glossing effect on hair, but are relatively high in carbohydrates and contain sugar. Fresh fruits should be included in the diet, but should be consumed in moderation. Wheat germ, the protein wonder-worker, is excellent for a good hair diet. Protein powders and brewer's yeast give additional helpful hair benefits.

Permissible snacks are: raw celery, cucumbers, radishes, hard cheese, pecans or walnuts, sugar-free chewing gum, and berries (strawberries, blueberries, etc.).

Snacks and foods to avoid are: sugar-base chewing gum, relishes, sweet pickles, cream soups (made from a flour base), yoghurt (extremely high in carbohydrates), syrups of any type, refined sugar (substitute small amounts of honey, raw sugar, or sugar substitutes).

Foods to absolutely reject as too high in sugar content and/or carbohydrates are: pasta, bread, stuffing, rice, soft drinks, watermelon, candy, catsup, and tomato paste products.

Avoid diuretics as they remove valuable minerals from the body and can prove very dangerous.

Shiny hair does not necessarily mean blooming health; however, most doctors agree that people with dull hair do have a greater tendency toward illness. Since hair problems can stem from illness, be sure to consult with your family physician for treatment. He is professionally qualified to get to the root of your illness and any accompanying hair problems.

Vitamins

Since certain vitamins are extremely beneficial to the hair, under some circumstances a doctor may recommend vitamins as a dietary supplement. Of the many vitamins, vitamin A is one of the most valuable hair vitamins. The best sources of vitamin A are animal foods such as liver, fish oils, or egg yolks, butter and cream. Studies show that when this vitamin is undersupplied to the body, hair becomes dry, lacking sheen and luster. Dandruff often accompanies this condition. In a 1954 publication of the University of Chicago Press, Flesch reports that deficiencies in vitamin A, riboflavin, biotin, inositol, pantothenic acid, pyridoxine, and vitamin E undoubtedly impair hair growth.

Deficiencies of at least four B vitamins, PABA, biotin, inositol, and pantothenic acid, appear to affect hair color. These deficiencies may lead to gray hair. Although hair color is rarely restored permanently by taking B vitamins, through following a healthy diet rich in all of the B vitamins, indications are that it may be possible to restore natural hair color at least temporarily.

Brewer's yeast is a key source of vitamin B complex. Experiments also show that substantial hair loss occurs in animals whose diets lack certain amino acids or are deficient in any one of the several B vitamins.

In 1946 a British investigator named Hughes concluded that a deficiency of the B vitamins, riboflavin, and pantothenic acid is the cause of straight hair. Another tip comes from Doctors Andrews and Domonkox, two well-known skin specialists associated with the Columbia Presbyterian Medical Center in New York. According to their findings, vitamin B complex and all the B vitamins, B_1, B_3, B_6, B_{12}, biotin, pantothenic acid), riboflavin, and nicotinamide aid in combatting serious forms of dandruff.

With all that has been written about the B vitamins, there are those about which relatively little is known. One of these is biotin, a vitamin now undergoing closer study. Although it has been known for some time that yeast offers the richest source of biotin, new investigations reveal that animals lacking biotin in their diet experience a number of negative reactions including substantial or complete loss of hair. Another B vitamin normally assumed to be adequately supplied by a proper diet is para-aminobenzoic acid, commonly called PABA. Initially, PABA rose to minor fame as an antigray-hair vitamin, since black animals when lacking this vitamin were known to turn gray. In experiments with human subjects carried out by Dr. Benjamin Sieve, it was noted that 70 percent of the people given 200 milligrams of PABA after each meal showed restoration of their natural hair color.

Although the B vitamin inositol has not undergone extensive studies, there are indications that this vitamin, too, has an effect on hair. Liver and yeast are good sources of this vitamin, as are wheat germ, whole-wheat bread, oatmeal, corn, and unrefined molasses. Studies show that when animals are purposely placed on diets which lack inositol, their hair falls out. When the vitamin is returned to the diet, the hair grows in again. By comparison, studies demonstrated that male animals lost their hair twice as fast as female animals, possibly indicating that the males treated required a higher ratio of inositol in their diet. As a result of these studies, inositol is often recommended by doctors as a dietary vitamin supplement for men who are experiencing hair loss or even baldness. In some cases, new hair growth has been reported in as little as a month's time.

Increasing the amount of any vitamin over that which is needed by the body, however, may result in unpleasant, perhaps dangerous side effects. To B or not to B? To be completely certain, consult with your physician; he will decide if you are lacking any one of the hair vitamins and can recommend the proper vitamin units for corrective purposes.

A HEALTHY DIET MEANS HEALTHY HAIR

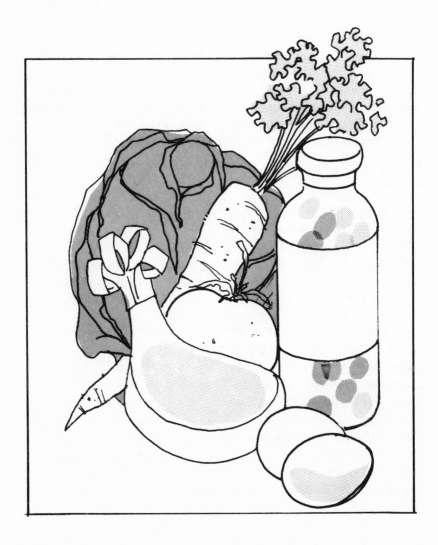

4.
Hereditary Factors

A Parisian physician, Dr. Pruener-Bey, once categorized hair into three separate types: straight, wavy, and wooly, which he attributed to heredity. Until recently, the ethnological weight which he gave hair remained relatively important for both liberals and intellectuals alike. Many still adhere to Dr. Pruener-Bey's ideas. However, we now realize that hair differences have little importance when compared to overwhelming hair similarities. That humanity has persisted in maintaining and enlarging upon its hairy differences seems pointless when the facts are examined. None of Dr. Pruener-Bey's information has been altered. "Straight" hair hangs naturally long and lank, straight as a ruler. It is completely free of waves, ripples, or curls. Under very strong magnification, a straight-hair strand resembles a standard strand of spaghetti at least as far as its shape is concerned. The cross section of either appears almost perfectly rounded. Color is nearly always black. Straight, long, lank hair is characteristic of Chinese, Mongol, and American Indians. "Wavy" hair is smooth or curly; its texture varies from

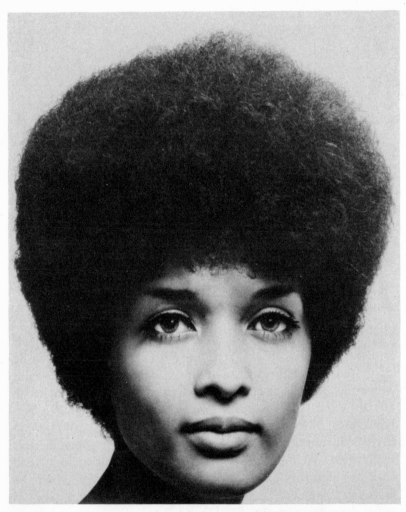

Wooly hair is short, crisp hair. Courtesy of Clairol Inc.

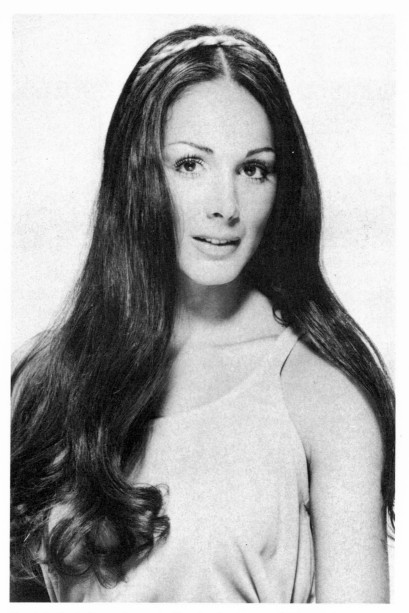

Straight hair hangs long and lank. Courtesy of Clairol Inc.

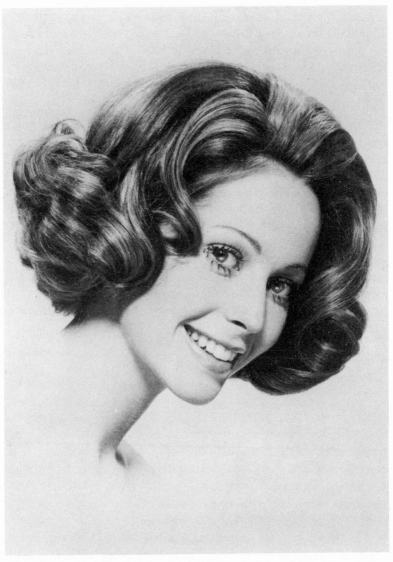

For maximum bounce, keep hair within short cut styles. Courtesy of Clairol Inc.

baby fine to semicoarse. Under intense magnification, the shape of a wavy-hair strand resembles tagliatelle, an ovular linguini strand. Wavy-hair colors run the gamut from fair extremely blond shades to dark brown and black. Wavy hair has its roots of origin in Europe and is characteristic of the Caucasian race. "Wooly" denotes short, crisp hair; also referred to as kinky, because kinks are generally formed as a result of the hair's tightness of curl. The color of wooly hair is almost always jet black. Under heavy magnification, the wooly-hair strands bear close resemblance to the strands of a flat linguini, although the hair strand is sometimes slightly more rounded. Hair can be fine, coarse, or of medium texture. Wooly hair is characteristic of the black races with the exception, for some reason, of a handful of natives in India and Australia. There are two basic varieties of wooly hair. In the first, the hair is relatively long, and curls are relatively large, which gives the head an appearance of being generously covered. In the second, the hair grows in very short, tight curls, which form little tufts surrounded by spaces that appear to be bare. The head looks as if it were dotted with pepperseed and, therefore, is sometimes referred to as peppercorn growth.

More Classified Information

Red hair is a happening strictly associated with freckles. There are technically no red-headed races.

The link between hair's classification and its absolute or relative length is about the same regardless of sex. Of the three groupings, straight hair is obviously longest, while wooly is shortest; wavy hair bridges the gap between the two. In any race, the lengths to which a man is physically capable of growing hair scarcely differs from what is femininely possible; Chinese pigtails or Indian braids being ample examples. Among pale faces, the hip-long-haired look is definitely in for both men and women, and blacks of either sex sport Afros, Afro Shags, or freedom cuts with equal success.

Today the report seems to be a case of merely splitting hairs. All the hairy differences that have been expounded upon over the years barely fit on the head of a pin. Factually, hair is hair, regardless of race, age, or sex. The importance allotted to its texture fails to consider that on any given scalp more than one texture of hair can and does exist. Hair at the temples or nape of the neck may have a tendency to curl; at the top, to be straight and sparse; by comparison, the sides may seem wavy and thick. The importance placed on straight and on curly hair seems much ado about nothing. The straightened hair of a black individual resembles that of any other race; it may be thin, thick, oily, dry, or whatever. Conversely, tightly curled hair, whether a birthright or artificially cultivated, behaves in a like manner in either case. Variations in the handling of hair are simply individual matters related to individual tastes based on a preference for a look or image.

Regardless of any other factor, problems concerning amount of curl (too little or too much), hair's density (thickness or thinness), and hair's general state are universal problems. Like leprosy, the phenomena of graying, thinning, balding, dry, or oily scalps are conditions which cannot be escaped by virtue of race; they may be lessened or intensified but that is all. Blacks, for example, suffer to a lesser degree from the problems of balding. Asians suffer least from the phenomenon of graying. In neither case is there total escape; problems are relative. Since hair is always hair, the principles of care remain ever constant for all peoples at all times. The fact is there's but a mere shred of difference between hair types.

5.
Drugs –
Their Effects on Hair

According to recent surveys, there may be twenty million pot smokers in America, not to mention countless others who are users of harsh or hard drugs. Regardless of anything you may have heard, read, or hoped, many drugs—including marijuana, hashish, LSD, Methedrine, the amphetamines, cocaine, heroin, and the barbiturates—do have specific pharmacological effects on the internal system of the body, and on both hair and scalp. Professional hair-dressers claim they can tell by the hair's texture, wet or dry, if someone has been taking drugs—even antibiotics. Hair seems less bouncy—less alive. Birth-control pills, diet pills, and tranquilizers can make the hair come out in handfuls.

In addition to any scalp effects, drugs have a marked effect on the nervous system, often leading to such characteristic symptoms as headaches, dizziness, loss of balance, tremors, twitching, anxiety, and depression, as well as physical changes including increased blood pressure, heart palpitations, inflamed blood vessels of the eyes, blurred vision, and swelling of the eyelids. The stomach and intestines may also be affected, resulting in vomiting, nausea, or diarrhea. Although danger signs are not always apparent, there is no doubt that abuse of drugs produces internal damage.

Some users say marijuana makes tensions disappear, therefore it's good for your head. Regardless of any other considerations, the fact is that the side effects of heavy pot smoking are physically injurious to the hair of any head.

Innumerable cases reported by doctors throughout the country clearly point up the fact that in many instances drugs are detrimental to the health of hair and skin. Reports in medical journals continually cite classic cases of individuals who have sought medical help because of severe hair loss, excessive dandruff, and blotching skin conditions, and who, during the course of treatment, have admitted to use of pot, LSD, or amphetamines. Even heavy smoking of regular cigarettes cuts down circulation. In cases where the patients switched from habitual drug use to a program of habitual hair care under professional surveillance, hair loss stopped and dandruff disappeared. It should also be noted that in addition to drug abuse, the patient's life style may also have contributed to hair and skin problems.

As a side issue, doctors working in free clinics around the country when interviewed agreed that the youthful counter-culture with its close communal living, sharing of clothing and beds, and poor hygienic conditions was giving the louse a new lease on life. Head lice are most common amongst people with long hair. A British scientist estimated that the best part of a million of his countrymen were infested with head lice.

Engulfed in drug-oriented surroundings, one may be just too dopey to worry about such necessities as clean hair, hygiene, vitamins, good nutrition, and self-respect. It seems apparent that apart from the damage drugs are capable of doing to the body, they may also produce an unhealthy psychological dependence. Only when a straight healthy mind exists can a healthy body be properly maintained under a great head of healthy hair. The only *H* to which anyone should ever become addicted is *Hair!*

6.
Female Hair Loss –
The Pill, Pregnancy and Hormones

Since hair and scalp mirror the body's state of health, thinning or loss of hair may be indications of a hormonal imbalance or disturbance. The Pill is often responsible for either condition, especially when birth control is discontinued. But when and where the Pill is involved, any unhappy hair results are almost always temporary with normal hair growth sure to follow.

Like the Pill, pregnancy may also result in hormonal imbalance, thereby causing hair to shed. Hair loss may be especially noticeable after childbirth, due to loss of the placenta and the huge hormonal output of the ovaries. Marked thinning of hair during postpregnancy is of a temporary nature and usually compensates for itself within a year. If a woman has any other form of hair loss, each pregnancy will help to stabilize it. After each childbirth she will normally rebound to the point where she would have been had she continued to lose hair gradually.

Besides the Pill or pregnancy, hair loss is sometimes attributed to hormone deficiency. This may call for replacement therapy. In this treatment, high doses of female hormones are given. This is why some women who take the Pill, which is high in female hormones, find it has beneficial side effects for hair. Estrogen seems to be helpful in stabilizing the balding process. (Taken in large doses, estrogen may cause regrowth of hair but should be taken only under a doctor's care because most of the side reactions are pelvic in nature.) Much depends upon whether the loss of hair is real or merely represents a resting phase of growing hair. If growing hairs are truly lost, baldness may indeed follow.

Sometimes, rather than a hormone deficiency, an excess of a hormone exists. Androgen, a male hormone, is an occasional offender. After menopause there is a gradual suppression of the female sex hormone, estrogen, because of a waning of glandular activity. In some women it is believed that the male hormone androgen may begin to exert its influence. In such cases, the woman has an internal glandular setup similar to that of her spouse and baldness may develop if the tendency runs in her side of the family. This is why baldness following the menopause is usually diagnosed as androgenic hair loss. Here again, a doctor will most likely prescribe replacement therapy. Another male hormone, testosterone, will, if present in large amounts, tend to make women lose their hair.

Sometimes at about fifty years of age, women experience thinning hair which often resembles the male type of baldness. In women, however, hair loss is more diffuse or scattered over the entire scalp. Hair loss, it appears, stems from a combination of heredity and glandular factors, especially since the human body manufactures both male and female sex hormones, an imbalance of which will register in changed hair production.

For women who suffer from seasonal fallout and don't know what to do, hormones again may help. Medically, it has been proven possible to suppress seasonal hair loss with estrogens; however, unless the amount of seasonal hair loss is substantial —you can lose up to 30 percent of your hair without its being considered a clinical loss—dermatologists will not normally take any action which involves hormones. Most agree that it is foolish to try to thwart the loss of hair that occurs naturally since, all in all, estrogens make very little cosmetic difference. In exceptional instances where the hair is unusually thin to begin with and is afflicted further by seasonal loss, high doses of estrogen may make the cosmetic difference; thus, in extreme cases, doctors may prescribe estrogen to diminish or stop further hair loss.

Despite hormonal therapy, the general medical consensus is that maintaining normal health and nutrition is the best ammunition against hair loss.

7.
Male Hair Loss and Testosterone

Has modern science come up with anything new to help reverse the process of male balding?

Before an answer can be given, it is necessary to know the kind of baldness involved. There are two types: hereditary baldness, seen most commonly in men, but sometimes affecting women; and alopecia areata, which can happen at any age in either sex. This latter type begins in small bald spots which expand and sometimes cover the whole scalp. The condition seems to be caused by inflammation of the connective tissue around the tiny blood vessels of the scalp. Sometimes this type can be helped by corticosteroid drugs, but the side effects may be even worse than the bald spots.

In the much more common male-pattern baldness, the hair doesn't literally fall out; it gradually becomes thin, stunted, and finally just disappears. The slowdown follows a characteristic horseshoe pattern on the scalp. Usually some visible hair is left on the sides and back of the head.

New Hope for Hair through the Male Sex Hormone Testosterone

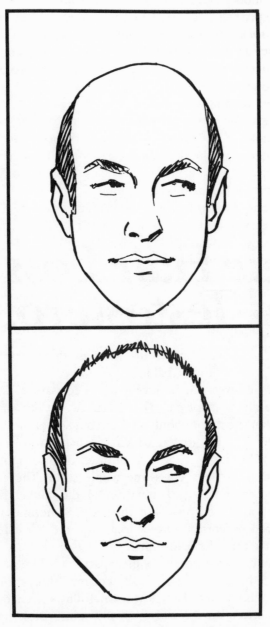

For male-pattern baldness, although results are not yet conclusive, modern science does offer new hope.

In an experiment reported in the *Journal of the American Medical Association,* Dr. Christopher M. Papa, while completing his residency in dermatology at the University of Pennsylvania, reported success in restoring hair in male-pattern baldness. He was able to grow hair on the heads of 16 out of 21 bald men, and at the presentation before the American Academy of Dermatologists he produced photographs to back up his claims. Although none of his successes had to be rushed to the barbers, there was definitely hair—in some cases long, coarse hair typical of that produced by a normal, thriving scalp. Said Dr. Papa, "We believe that baldness is reversible."

The technique used by Dr. Papa and his associate, Dr. A. M. Klingman, is simple. It consists in applying a cream containing a male hormone, testosterone, to the scalp once a day—in this instance over a five-month period. The success of testosterone is a paradox, since all hair specialists agree that an excess of testosterone in the male system is an important factor in causing baldness. "Perhaps this fact has up to now caused other researchers to shy away from testosterone," said Dr. Papa, who made his own discovery quite accidentally while doing research on the process of aging in skin.

Dr. Papa found that hair regrew only where the cream was rubbed on. This led him to conclude that the cream had a direct local pharmacological effect only on the underlying scalp cells rather than on the body in general. Viewed under a microscope, the supportive cells of the hair follicles seemed to have re-captured their youth. Fuzzy hairs, usually visible on a bald head only when magnified, were visibly transformed in about 10 percent of the scalp area into long, stout, terminal hairs. It appeared that the longer the treatment, the better the results. One man who had been on the program for a year showed a 25 percent response. It was shown that testosterone does not lead to the creation of any new follicles on a bald scalp, but apparently does stimulate hair growth in those that remain.

Dr. Papa's patients, ages 29 to 78, were residents of a home for the aged and inmates of a county prison; therefore, they could be closely observed and given frequent examinations. Since testosterone is a powerful substance, it is only applied when the patient can be kept under close surveillance. Testosterone can aggravate certain heart conditions and cause other complications.

It must, therefore, be emphasized that hormone cream containing testosterone may not be the final answer to hereditary male-pattern baldness, but at least there is hope. If and when more extensive research is carried on, for many there may be a cure. Dr. Papa, although sympathetic about baldness, is not personally interested in continuing with further research since this was not his original endeavor. Hopefully, however, his discovery will stimulate others to pick up where he left off.

8.
Coping With Hair and Scalp Conditions

When was the last time someone complimented your hair? If you can't remember or don't want to think back that far, then it is high time you took another look in the mirror. For as long as you can recollect, you've probably been giving your head the treatment—spraying, styling, coloring, permanenting, straightening. teasing, doing everything under the sun to it with no thought as to timing. Untimely combinations of treatments do more harm than good! It is reassuring to know, however that even when the damage is done, you can get your hair back to virgin state by cutting off the lightened, straightened, permanented, dyed, or what-have-you hair, after it has sufficiently grown out.

New York cosmotologist and hair expert Guy Paris, in charge of research at Paris West Hairstylists, offers this summation for our common hair problems. Often, he says, we put beauty before health by rolling, teasing, and torturing our hair with bleaches, coloring agents, lotions, and so-called conditioners, all of which are specially concocted to bring about rapid and drastic chemical changes and which in fact ultimately affect the very structure of hair. In the end, hair loss, split ends, dryness, and unmanageability bring us right back to more chemical treatments and further hair abuse. Bad timing and lack of knowledge are the culprits in this vicious circle.

Now is the time to analyze where your well-meaning efforts went wrong and what you can do to set your locks right again. Remember, conditions like dull, dry, itchy scalp; oily, unruly hair; split ends; damaged or thinning hair are problems common to both men and women. About the only problem a man escapes is the nightly ritual of setting his hair before going to bed—which, perhaps, is compensated for each morning. Regardless of your hair problems, help is available. With modern techniques and products replacing age-old misconceptions and outdated remedies, no one need ever hide his or her head in shame. Proper diagnosis and treatment is available.

Microscopic analysis such as performed at Paris West Hairstylists ends speculation. Before-and-after, on-the-spot microanalysis shows factual improvement as opposed to fanciful guesswork.

More often than not, righting the wrongs is only a matter of rebalancing the hair's chemistry. When this is done, hair and scalp are put back to normal in quick order. Under correct diagnosis, oily hair can be de-oiled, thinning hair can be fattened, and flaky scalps can be deflaked. It's even conceivable that a balding spot can bloom again. To begin coping with correction requires: (1) pinpointing the problems; (2) treating the causes (usually as simple as discontinuing the evils of past ways); and (3) giving top priority to a faithful program of daily hair care. Persistent neglect of any hair or scalp problem results only in adding to existing problems. To have great hair requires consistent care. Forget past rationalizations. A magnificent head of beautiful hair is not an accident of birth; it's the sum total of proper care, getting in on all the newest improvements, and never saying die.

To classify the condition of your hair, shampoo and dry as you would normally. Wait forty-eight hours; then, in front of a well-lit mirror, examine your hair carefully. Check the hair ends in various sections all over your head. Study the color, luster, and texture. Touch your hair from root to ends; then evaluate your hair type according to the descriptions outlined here.

Normal Hair

Everyone's goal is normal hair. Hair has beautiful sheen, great gloss, and good elasticity. Scalp is clear. Color is great. If this description fits your hair and scalp—congratulations, at the moment you're free of high-level hassles!

Dry Hair

Dry hair breaks easily, is brittle, lacks sheen and elasticity; ends may be broken or fuzzy. Scalp is tight and often flaky. Hair is snarly when wet.

Cause: Dry hair can result from using the wrong type of shampoo, improper rinsing, careless bleaching, overteasing, too frequent permanents, or too much exposure to the sun.

Correction: Stop any of the above mentioned practices and start your new approach. Dry hair and scalp require a program of regular lubrication to combat the lack of moisture and natural lubricants. Lubricants will also help to strengthen weakened dry hair. This is true regardless of whether dryness is a natural state or one caused by overprocessing. Use of an instant protein conditioner will get to the root of your problems as well as to any weakened or dry ends. Once a month, take time for a cream conditioner. Allow the cream conditioner to remain on the hair for twenty to thirty minutes. To intensify the treatment, wrap a towel around your head and use a special heat cap. If the tips of your hair appear frizzy, try working a cream hair dressing into the ends. Since dry hair has a definite tendency to be lusterless, do not shampoo more than necessary. Make certain that the conditioners and lubricants you use at home do not require three or four soapings before they are removed from the hair, as this negates your efforts. For example, if hot castor oil is used, it will take at least four to five washings before the oil slick will disappear. Despite your castor oil treatment, your hair will remain dry and lusterless, due to overshampooing. Here are three oil recipes to liven dry hair and improve the condition of your scalp.

Hot Oil Treatment

Heat vegetable or baby oil to a comfortable temperature; massage into scalp and hair. Dip a towel in hot water; wring partially dry; wrap around hair. When towel begins to cool, replace with another hot towel. Continue treatment for twenty minutes. Shampoo well.

Overnight Oil Treatment

For renewed sheen and luster, rub dry hair with linseed oil before going to bed. Be sure to wrap your head in a plastic shower cap to protect pillow and sheets. For glowing results, shampoo first thing in the morning.

Aid to Dry, Color-Treated Hair

Stroke cotton soaked in warm olive oil through hair, starting about four inches from the scalp to hair ends. Place your head in a heat cap and let your hair steep for about fifteen minutes. Next, shampoo it once, dry, and then again wet, Rinse and rinse.

When shampooing, water should be kept warm, not hot. Use a nondetergent shampoo to remove soil and hair spray effectively while leaving the hair soft and flexible. Cream rinses will also help curb static electricity. If you are in the habit of using a home dryer, dab the ends of your hair with a cream hairdressing before setting your hair. Many hairdressers will massage a conditioner over the entire head of hair before setting. You, too, can do this at home, as well as in between shampoos to add extra sheen to your hair. In opposition to general belief, hair dryers do not dry out the hair's natural oils. The only thing a dryer dries out is the water your towel can't squeeze out. Be sure to set your dryer at warm—not hot. Daily massage and brushing will help to carry the natural scalp oils—your own personal conditioning agents—to dry tips. At least twice each day, rotate your fingertips over the scalp for approximately five minutes. This will help to stimulate the natural scalp oils. Always protect dry hair from winter wind and strong sun by wearing a hat or scarf. Only through a program of constant care will you be able to trade in your dry, dull locks for shiny beautiful hair.

Dull Hair

Dull hair lacks luster and sheen and is often dry, a common problem among males.

Cause: This condition may be caused by dryness or by improper shampoo and rinsing techniques.

Correction: If dullness is driving you to distraction, take heed. Follow the conditioning treatments outlined for dry hair; conditioners are the quickest means of putting shine back in your hair. The reason men suffer from dull-hair problems to a greater degree than do women is undoubtedly due to the fact that men are great believers in daily showers and usually wind up using soap on both the hair and scalp, as well as on their bodies. Although soap and water may not negatively affect the body, the alkaline content in soap does have a drying effect on the hair. Executive heads, it seems, do not always comprehend the value of utilizing proper shampoo preparations. Hair may be washed as often as necessary, providing a nondetergent shampoo is used. It is important to rinse the hair thoroughly and frequently to avoid any leftover shampoo residue, as this is sure to dull the hair. Shampoo film, unfortunately, is sometimes a hazard of hard water. If the water in your area is hard, try adding a teaspoon of baking soda to the final rinse water. This will help to eliminate residue and overcome any dullness caused by hard water.

Oily Hair

Oily hair occurs less frequently than dry hair. Hair is lifeless, dull, limp; looks stringy. The scalp and hair show oil deposits within a day or two after shampooing. Hair at forehead, part, temples, and nape of neck are especially affected. Dandruff frequently is part of the problem.

Cause: An oily condition is often a natural state. Lack of air or sun, or the wrong type of shampoo will act as aggravators.

Correction: For the most part, dermatologists prescribe more shampooing. Use of a specially formulated shampoo at least twice a week helps make oily hair look alive. The object is never to let your hair look like it needs to be washed. Often, a simple drying shampoo will control the problem. After shampooing, a conditioner should be used to help fluff up the hair. There are numerous cream rinses available which are intended especially for oily hair. As a starter, try one of the conditioners that must be left on the scalp for one full minute before being rinsed out. Always rinse with tepid water first and then with cold water. There are also new oil-blotting rinses on the market which aid in the removal of excess oil and help to prolong the period between shampoos. Once a month, try one of the deep-penetration conditioners which must be left on the hair for twenty to thirty minutes before being rinsed out with tepid water. To keep oily hair looking bright between shampoos, use an instant aerosol shampoo to aid in absorbing any excess oil. First spray on the dry shampoo and then fluff up the hair with your fingers. Use a clean natural-bristle hairbrush and stroke hair gently until the instant shampoo is completely brushed out. To keep bristles at top-level performance, in between brush strokes, rub your hairbrush over a terry-cloth towel. If an instant shampoo is not handy, dab a ball of cotton moistened with cologne or astringent at scalp areas where oil collects.

If oily hair is limp or stringy, make use of one of the body-building conditioners which will help to improve hair texture, or try using a conditioner with a built-in setting lotion. A hair dryer will help to air out oily hair. Natural fresh air and sunshine will aid in clearing up oiliness, too.

Oily hair should be kept at midneck length, rather than long. A midneck length assimilates scalp oils better and keeps hair looking fluffier longer.

When and if external methods do not improve an oily hair and scalp condition, your dermatologist may offer internal therapy by prescribing an estrogen drug to cut down on the body's oil-producing activities. Persons with oily hair and scalp have the hope of knowing that though oiliness may be a problem now, the problem diminishes naturally as one grows older.

Half-Dry—Half-Oily Hair

With half-dry—half-oily hair, scalp may be oily but oil does not carry to the ends of the hair strands. Ends are dry and uncontrollable, and breakage often occurs.

Cause: Half-dry—half-oily hair, although sometimes a natural state, is more often the result of using a shampoo that is simply too drying for dry hair and scalp areas. Insufficient brushing agitates and aggravates the condition.

Correction: To control dry, unruly ends, trim the hair. Do not shampoo more than is necessary, as overshampooing tends to aggravate the dry, unruly areas of your hair. Between shampoos, spray a dry shampoo on oily areas and then brush away. Give hair a deep-conditioning treatment after each shampoo. Allow the conditioner to remain on the hair fifteen to thirty minutes—preferably once a week or, at a minimum, every other week. When curling the hair, use a body-building conditioner or setting lotion. Between shampoos, add extra manageability to your hair by working a cream hairdressing conditioner into the ends of the hair. To add sheen without making the hair look oily, use one of the spray conditioners. Remember to brush the hair daily in order to distribute oil from the scalp to dry hair ends. This will help improve both the oily areas as well as the dry areas. By getting the dry areas oilier and the oily areas drier, you will solve the present doldrums. It is all that simple.

Fine Hair, Limp Hair

With fine, limp hair, hair strands are lightweight, often matted looking. Hair itself may be dry or oily. Styling presents untold difficulties.

Cause: Fine hair may be a natural condition or the result of an improper diet. The wrong haircut will make fine hair even more unmanageable.

Correction: Fine hair is not necessarily more prone to oil, it only shows the effects of oil more quickly and drastically than other hair types. Fine hair looks twice as full and bouncy right after shampooing. When selecting a shampoo for fine hair, choose one that corresponds to your hair type, be it dry, oily, or normal. Avoid cream rinses that tend to soften the hair; instead, pick one of the new instant protein conditioners which aids in giving the hair extra body and manageability. Gels and setting lotions with extra holding ingredients will also help control baby-fine hair. If your hair is fine, but otherwise normal, try a mild body permanent for extra support. When setting, do not wind rollers too tightly or fine hair will end up looking frizzy and unruly. Fine or limp hair requires a good haircut. A blunt cut, one cut straight across, will tend to make fine hair look fuller. For maximum bounce, keep hair within

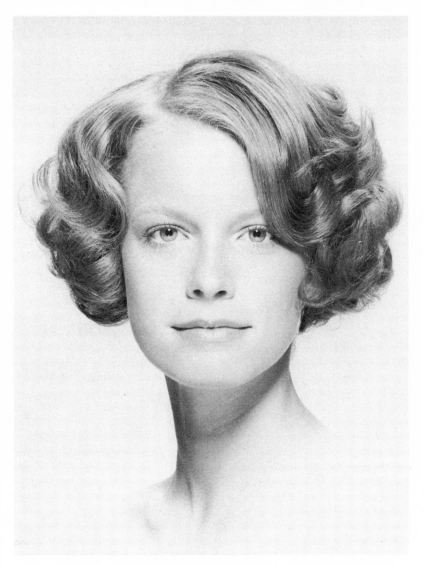

Fine, thin or sparse hair responds better to short, fluffy styles that help make hair look fuller. Courtesy of Clairol Inc.

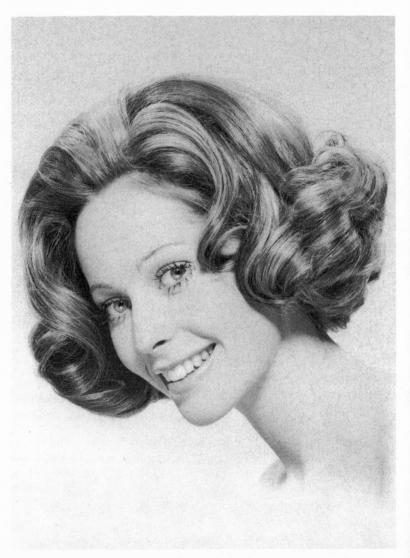

Hair at the temples or nape of the neck may have a tendency
to curl; at the top, to be straight and sparse; by comparison,
the sides may seem wavy and thick. Courtesy of Clairol Inc.

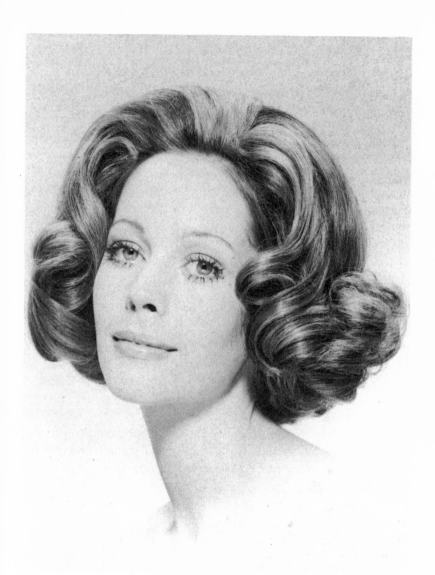

The appeal of a woman's hair is a matter of texture, color, movement and even scent. Courtesy of Clairol Inc.

short-cut styles. To give fine hair the extra firm foundation it needs, section the hair narrowly and very lightly back-comb. For additional control, add a touch of hair spray and perhaps a sheen hairdressing. Fine hair should be brushed lightly each day to reduce any possible hair spray buildup. It is important that hair and scalp be kept scrupulously clean. The minute your hair looks matted, corrective steps are necessary.

Jean-Louis Hym of Cinandre, in New York City, has an unusual remedy for thin hair: a henna rinse. Henna is an organic pigment that ordinarily tints hair red, but can be obtained in treated form so that coloring properties are removed. *Both* kinds of henna add body and a look of greater volume to hair. Medium brunettes can use regular henna for bright, auburn highlights; blondes and those with black hair should keep to the treated kind to avoid artificial-looking color. Avoid permanenting or straightening. Such processes are ineffective on henna-rinsed hair and may, in certain cases, be harmful.

Wiry, Coarse Hair

Wiry, coarse hair is stiff, unmanageable, excessively bulky, often overly curly. Hair tends to frizz.

Cause: Wiry hair is most often a natural hereditary condition. Usually an underactive thyroid is to blame and reflects in coarse hair. When wiry, coarse hair is not properly shaped, hair appears even bulkier.

Correction: The best controller for a bushy head of hair is frequent cutting and shaping. Any unnecessary bulk should be thinned, although thinning can make hair difficult to manage. Plan to visit an expert stylist or barber; don't go to just any cut-rate clip joint. What you save, you may pay for later.

A cap of chic all-over curls generally looks best and behaves better naturally. A feathered cut with a layered nape offers maximum manageability. To control your hair and achieve a clean contour, apply a setting lotion and comb thoroughly through the hair. When setting hair, use giant rollers to attain a smooth uncluttered line. *Avoid any experimentation with home hair straighteners.* If you feel your hair must be straightened, let a professional handle it. A cream rinse after shampooing will make coarse hair softer to the touch and easier to manage. Top off with moisture-resistant or antihumidity spray to keep uptight hair from kinking or frizzing. Between shampoos a little pomade or hairdressing smoothed on will help to hold hair in line and will add glistening highlights.

Damaged Hair

Damaged hair is brittle and porous; breaks easily; usually is limp and without elasticity. It tangles badly when wet, and may be brassy if bleached.

Cause: Badly damaged hair is largely, if not solely, due to gross mistreatment. Overtinting, bleaching, lightening, over-exposure to sun, too frequent permanents, or straightening processes are generally to blame. Add to this, brushing fine hair too vigorously, careless combing of teased hair, overteasing, and general overmanipulation. Sleeping on rollers is particularly harmful; the friction created when taut hair is pulled between rollers and a bed pillow can easily tear and break off weakened hair strands. Wire mesh, stiff brush, or clip-on type rollers are brutal to the hair.

Correction: First and foremost, discontinue any of the damaging practices in which you are now engaged. If your hair is seriously damaged, seek professional help quickly—the initial reconditioning your hair needs is too complicated to do success-fully at home, and trying to cure your damaged hair problems yourself would more than likely cause additional grief. Dam-aged hair needs professional products, professional care, and the help of a professional hairdresser. Any reliable hairdresser will automatically propose a program of intensive hair care lasting for two or three weeks, and will no doubt insist that you give your hair a rest from any of the chemicals you have been using. A typical salon treatment includes gentle shampoo or a professional deep-conditioning treatment, often with a heating cap to intensify conditioning, and scalp massages. Only after having received professional help can you properly help your condition at home. If you are using a hair spray, shampoo the spray out as soon as possible so your hair will not break off. After the home shampoo, blot your hair dry with a towel; then dry it very, very gently. Don't rub your hair vigorously or brush it dry. Use a conditioner which is left on after shampooing and which will strengthen your hair by penetrating and plumping up the weakened hair shafts.

If you use a home hair dryer, avoid the hot cycle. When styling, do not pull or tug the hair. Use only a wide-toothed comb and a natural-bristle brush. Metal combs or brushes can harm your hair two ways: (1) metals transmit static electricity to your hair; and (2) a metal brush or comb is always either hotter or cooler than the air. The cold fluctuation of a metal comb touching your hair expands or shrinks hair cells and therefore weakens or breaks off precious strands. Steer clear of overbrushing and overteasing. Brutal yanking or pulling at the scalp will create excess tension and cause weak hair to snap and break off. To avoid the hazards of sleeping on rollers, hairdressers advise women to set their hair before going to bed. A hair dryer set on a warm cycle should be used. When your hair is dry, remove the curlers and clips, but do not comb out. A hair net placed over the head will hold your hair in place while you sleep. Another solution: Get up earlier and set your hair before your day begins. Whether you set your hair before retiring or in the early morning hours, either plan will spare your hair from the damage caused by sleeping on rollers.

Additional information — metal hairpins and bobby pins are coated with an acrylic substance which at least for a while protects the hair from splits and breakage. Once the acrylic substance is worn off the tips, this usually means three weeks after you buy pins, throw the old ones out. Avoid rubber bands, they too tear and pull out hair. Use yarn or a tortoise shell interlocking comb. Avoid metals.

A last word of hope — troubled hair can always be cut an inch or two. If that doesn't do it, except perhaps in complete disaster cases, a wig can be worn until new hair growth replaces the old.

Split Ends (Thrichoptiloses)

Split ends are hairs split at the end in two or possibly three sections. Ends appear frizzy, dry, and discolored. This condition often accompanies damaged, dull, or dry hair.

Cause: Check your hairbrush and comb for possible rough tips that may be responsible for slicing your locks. Excess sun, permanent dyes or bleaches also contribute to the problem of split ends.

Correction: Trim away split ends so they do not make their way up the hair shaft to cause total damage to your hair. A shampoo specifically recommended for dry hair helps to combat dry ends. For added strength and sheen, follow shampoo with a one-minute protein conditioning treatment. Between shampoos massage hair dressing into the tips of the hair to help keep ends pliable. Be sure to brush hair gently and to keep trimming any dead ends away. Avoid teasing, metal curlers, brush rollers, uncoated bobby pins, or any sharp-edged barrettes. Before buying a new brush or comb, check to see that there are no sharp edges to endanger your hair. To avoid splitting or tearing the hair, take off any rings from your fingers before you massage or wash your hair. Some professionals counterattack split ends by resorting to the old European method of singeing: a technique which seals split ends and prevents the split from traveling up the hair shaft.

Guy Paris of Paris West Hairstylists, located at 157 West 72nd Street in New York City, has a unique antidote for Thrichoptiloses, i.e., befrizzled ends. Guy calls his technique organic flame cutting, which he says helps hair feel stronger and look more attractive; hair doesn't lose overall length in the process. Organic flame cutting goes one step further than the singeing technique of European beauticians. First, hair is treated with protein to condition and protect the outside sheath. Thereafter, as much hair as will go around a finger is twisted so that split, befrizzled ends pop away from the strand. At this stage Guy lightly singes away the split ends one by one via candle flame. According to Guy, if hair is brushed and properly lubricated and if it is not mistreated as in the past, split ends will not recur. Guy encourages and teaches effective home hair-care techniques and recommends use of organic products to help maintain the hair's proper acid/alkaline balance. Although weekly salon visits are not always necessary, Guy contends that hair and scalp must be professionally examined at periodic intervals if hair is to remain in top-notch condition.

Obviously, flame cutting is not a do-it-yourself venture. Also, if hair must be lightened or dyed, just as with singeing, the services of a reputable professional who will automatically condition your hair after each and every session are advisable.

Flaky Scalp

A flaky scalp is an unhealthy scalp condition, often confused with dandruff, which it is not.

Cause: Flaking of the scalp is a normal phenomenon since the human scalp, even at its healthiest, will show a mild degree of scaling. Like the rest of your skin, the scalp regularly sloughs off bits of its dead outer layer. The purpose of the external layer of scalp skin is to provide a tough, resilient barrier to protect the tissue below. Normally, your scalp's outermost layer is composed of twenty to forty layers of hardened, dead cells which are rubbed or worn off every day, a few layers at a time. As the outer layers go, they are replaced by new cells which keep the barrier intact. When the scalp is entirely healthy, this sloughing goes on unnoticed—the flakes being too small to cause attention. Excessive flaking is usually the result of a lack of humidity in the air, a dry scalp, improper rinsing, or a rundown physical condition.

Correction: To achieve a thick, silky head of hair, you must begin with a healthy scalp. Leading specialists claim that excessive hair loss and even baldness have more to do with an unhealthy scalp than with heridity. Your scalp is considered healthy when it feels loose to the touch and is free of noticeable scale, signs of dandruff or bacterial infection. The way to a healthy scalp is through cleanliness and a program of basic treatment: frequent shampooing, thorough rinsing, and extra brushing to stimulate and remove any loose, flaky particles from the scalp and hair. A nondrying shampoo is recommended. So is investing in a humidifier. Proper rest and a good diet are your reinforcements to gain or keep a healthy scalp. *Since flaking may be indicative of a serious scalp disorder, if improvements are not seen within two weeks, a visit to a dermatologist is in order.*

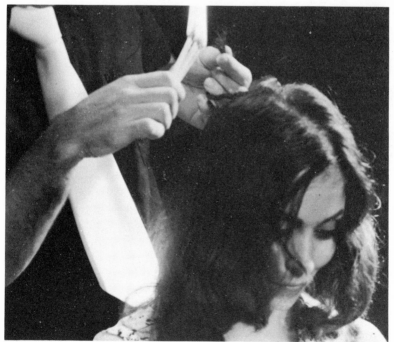

Guy of Paris West Hair Stylists in New York City makes split ends disappear, fine hair appear thicker without loss of length, with his flame cut.

9.
Corrective Measures

Falling flakes, falling hair, or departed hair are problems which descend upon many of us. Whether miniscule or massive, all three states require the closest of scrutiny.

Dandruff

The most common scalp ailment known, chiefly characterized by excessive scaling—leading to flakiness, itchiness, and embarrassment—is dandruff.

When normal scaling of the scalp speeds up to a point where you can no longer control it, you have dandruff. Instead of unnoticeable scaling, flakes may peel away twenty to fifty layers thick, often before the life cycle of the cells is finished. These flakes are plainly noticeable and are referred to as dandruff. The transition from normal scaling to excessive dandruff may be so gradual that it is difficult to determine where one condition ends and the other begins. Dandruff shows up in two varieties—the dry and the greasy. In severe dandruff cases, there may be hyperactivity or hypersecretion of the oil glands of the scalp, making the scalp oily. Extra sebaceous glands add an oil secretion to the dead scales. This combination, together with germs and dust from the air, forms dandruff flakes which only seem to be dry.

In a simple dandruff case there is no inflammation, swelling, redness, or overt infection. Any one of these signs points to something more serious than common dandruff. More than likely serious disorder exists, such as seborrheic dermatitis, psoriasis, or microbial scalp infection.

Medical authorities now consider dandruff, even the mild variety, as a disease. Clinically, dandruff is described as seborrhea capitos or excessive sebum production of the scalp. Based on recent research, it has been noted that in the past ten years dandruff problems have become more serious and more frequent. In the normal scalp, the process of sloughing off old cells and the manufacturing of their replacements is orderly and complete; while in the dandruff scalp, there is mass disorder and often the departing cells are not dead before leaving the scalp. Why there should be a speedup in the scalp's cell production remains a mystery. Contrary to popular theory, although bacteria may aggravate a dandruff condition, germs do not cause the initial problem.

Cause: As the precise cause of dandruff is unknown, there is no basis for assuming, as some advertisers do, that germs are the villains and antiseptic shampoos the good guys.

There appear to be two different causes—internal and external. Among the myriad of internal causes suspected are: hormonal imbalance, poor health, poor hygiene, allergic hypersensitivity, lack of rest, emotional stress, diet excesses involving sugar, fats, and starch, and lack of proper nutrition.

The most popular theory based upon an external cause is that dandruff is a mild form of disease caused by the presence of microorganisms like bacteria and fungi which inhabit the scalp. Although many authorities have supported this view, evidence to confirm the theory is missing. Tests on normal scalp skin and dandruff scalp skin have not shown any evidence of micro-organisms living within the scalp skin. If microorganisms are the cause of dandruff, they are probably an indirect cause. Chemical changes of the scalp or face may also be an external cause. Possibly microorganisms secretly manufacture a chemical that penetrates the skin; but scientists have yet to prove it. Nevertheless, most forms of antidandruff products are based on germ-killing ingredients. Ninety-four percent of all Americans aged twelve or older have had dandruff, have it now, or will have it sooner or later. It is not merely a seasonal occurrence as some people believe. It only appears to be more frequent during winter months, probably due to the wearing of darker clothing and hats and other types of headgear. Dandruff is equally common during warm-weather months. Whoever you are and wherever you live, you probably have at some time experienced some degree of dandruff. For most people, fortunately, dandruff is not long-lasting or of a serious nature. Yet a minimum of sixty-seven million dollars a year is spent by Americans for antidandruff shampoos, rinses, hairdressings, and prescriptions, while the mystery of what causes the problem remains unsolved.

Correction: If you're flaking out because of dandruff, take hope. There are a quantity of products at your disposal. Although there is no known cure, you can keep the problem from getting into your hair and under your skin. Even the severest case of dandruff can be controlled. Don't become discouraged if dandruff flakes recur. With proper attention, you will be able to eliminate the telltale signs almost as quickly as they develop. The idea is always to remain one step ahead of the problem, thereby maintaining constant control.

Do not allow a slight case of dandruff to grow worse. Combat dandruff by following a faithful routine of hair care, which includes daily brushing, massaging, and frequent shampooing—every three to five days—and, if your case warrants, proper medication.

Antidandruff or medicated shampoos work best. There are antidandruff shampoos available for both oily and dry hair conditions. Shampoo regularly. Once a week for dry hair, twice a week for oily. Before shampooing, brush your hair thoroughly; then massage the scalp until it tingles. Wet hair thoroughly. If your case of dandruff is heavy, use hot, hot water, the hottest your head can bear. Lather in shampoo. Use a small toothbrush to massage the scalp and to help lift the dandruff flakes away from your crown and into the suds. If you have sharp fingernails, be careful not to scratch your scalp, as this may dislodge live cells rather than the dead flaky ones. Rinse your scalp under a barrage of water, parting the hair in at least eight or nine areas, so that the water gets to all parts and rinses the scalp thoroughly clear of suds and flakes. Repeat the whole procedure a second time.

Thorough cleasning of the scalp and hair will keep dandruff flakes out of sight for up to three days. (It takes the scalp up to three days before it can generate a new batch of snowy flakes.) Of the multitude of commercial shampoos on the market, the mildest are coconut oil and a combination olive-oil and castile-soap formula. Although detergent shampoos will clean well, they very often cause dryness. If the scalp is oily, detergent shampoos are all right. For dandruff suffers, there are numerous popular-brand medicated shampoos—Enden, Banish, Head and Shoulders, Fostex, Rinse Away, Double Danderine—to name a few.

For very severe cases of dandruff, dermatologists normally prescribe ointment or lotion preparations containing sulphur, salicylic acid, resorcinol, tar, selenium sulfide, and cadmium sulfide. The concentration and frequency of use is dependent upon the severity of the case for which it is prescribed. Some prescription products, though excellent for the scalp, are tedious to use and unduly harsh on the hair. Prescription products should only be used while under the care of a doctor.

For normal everyday dandruff, drugstores carry a wide variety of medicinal preparations, shampoos, and hairdressings, available without a doctor's prescription. It is generally agreed that drugstore products which contain zinc pyritheone or selenium sulfide are the most effective in ridding the scalp of dandruff flakes. After-shampoo lotions or hairdressings containing quaternary ammonia work, too. There are differing opinions regarding the value of products containing sulfur, salicylic acid, and tar, although all three agents have been used for years in connection with dandruff. When purchasing new products, be sure to check out the ingredients.

Keep in mind that all flaking is not indicative of dandruff. If your scalp shows loose flakes but the skin beneath appears normal, all you may need is a little extra shampooing and a more frequent brushing routine. What is thought to be dandruff may also turn out to be just flakes of built-up powder substances caused by overuse of hair spray.

If your scalp shows signs of redness, swelling, scabbing, or gooeyness—accompanied by flakes—in all likelihood, you are being plagued by a scalp disease, possibly psoriasis or ringworm. Any one of the above symptoms requires the attention of a physician. Crusty dandruff accompanied by redness and inflammation of the scalp may be indicative of a condition called seborrheic dermatitis. In order to avoid the possibility of permanent damage to hair follicles. be sure to visit a dermatologist if your scalp shows either redness or swelling.

Many men live under the constant fear that dandruff may lead to baldness. Again, take hope. Although these conditions may occur simultaneously, there is absolutely no known cause-and-effect relationship between the two.

And for oily hair-dandruff worriers, be it known that there are untold numbers of cases of dandruff and oiliness lasting for years without leading to any abnormal hair thinning. If hair and scalp are oily and flaky, shampoo often—every other day, if necessary, and do not allow lotions or face creams to invade either the hairline or the hair itself.

Summary of Helpful Hints to Dandruff Sufferers

1. Brush and comb hair regularly. Use combs with rounded teeth and a soft natural-bristle brush.

2. Use hair cosmetics with caution. Read labels and follow directions carefully.

3. Live sensibly. Diet, rest, sleep, exercise, and lack of tensions are important for the well-being of your head and scalp.

4. Ideal antidandruff preparations should be nontoxic, simple to use, effective against itching and excessive oiliness. They should soften the scalp skin and be able to kill a wide range of bacteria and fungi.

5. Be aware that there are four varieties of antidandruff products available. Instead of being both doctor and patient, before combining products, visit a dermatologist for advice.

6. Shampoos, rinses, and preparations to use are:

   a. Detergent-dandruff remover—solution applied to the scalp five to twenty minutes prior to shampooing.

   b. Medicated shampoos—the most effective brands contain such active ingredients as sulfur, salicylic acid, resorcinol, or trademarked products such as Theone.

   c. After-shampoo rinses—these usually contain a quaternary ammonium compound to reduce scaling.

   d. Antiseptic scalp preparation—antiseptic lotions sometimes compounded as hairdressings which are applied to the scalp and contain such stimulants as tincture of capsicum, tincture of cantharides, chloral hydrate, and resorcinol monoacetate, etc.

The worst side effect of dandruff is sheer embarrassment. People turn off at the sight of snowy flakes on a blue serge suit or on a black dress. In this day and age, there is no worthy excuse for being unable to keep normal dandruff under control. By following a steady routine of good hygiene and daily care, no one should ever be left feeling flaky again.

Thinning (Falling) Hair

Noticeable hair loss, sparse hair, possible balding areas are symptoms of thinning or falling hair.

Hair grows in cycles, and departs normally in a systematic manner. Each hair grows at a rate of approximately one-third of a millimeter a day for two to six years, depending on your genes. In a three-month period, hair grows approximately one inch. After one-thousand days of growth, hair goes into a resting phase which lasts for roughly one-hundred days. As the growing phase starts up again, new hair is produced and the older resting hairs are shed by the wayside. Growth and natural loss are systematized so that at no time does your entire head of hair grow and rest simultaneously. Since man does not shed all of his hair at once, a normal individual does not lose hair density.

Researchers, experimenting over a five-year period testing seasonal hair loss, have found that November brings the highest amount of hair loss. Around May, hair loss begins diminishing. Although mammals may shed seasonally, humans shed periodically, usually at the ages of twenty-six, thirty-six, and fifty-four. If you are twenty-six and feel your hair is falling out, it probably is just a normal sign of overall hair exchange. If you have a crew cut, don't worry about the eighty-seven hairs you may be losing per day. If your hair is chin-length, a loss of sixteen hairs a day is normal. Girls with waist-length hair should not lose more than two hairs a day. If your hair is falling out. don't cut it off. Cutting the hair shorter only weakens roots and makes them shrink. thereby ruining the very foundation of your hair. For your information, hair can never grow more than eight feet—that's the limit.

It has already been established that in the northern hemisphere, summertime improves the growth of hair and reduces hair loss, but a noticeable thinning may actually take place due to hereditary factors or as the result of emotional strain, scalp infections, fatigue, or internal factors such as anemia, high fever, or malaria. A hyperthyroid condition is often reflected in sparse baby-fine hair. Women who have lost hair following their first childbirth, lose less with the second child and even less with a third child. It is the initial change of life style that apparently alters thyroid production. But after two or three children, apparently motherhood no longer represents monumental change and, therefore, the thyroid is not affected. Hair loss following childbirth occurs four months after delivery and lasts between two and eight weeks.

If you are healthy, free of emotional stress, and eat a well-balanced nourishing diet, no more than 5 percent of your hair will be in a rest phase at one time. If you are unhealthy, emotionally disturbed, or malnourished, your hair may be forced into a premature resting period, resulting in obvious hair loss.

Cause: Mistreatment can also be the cause of excessive hair loss. Pulling a comb roughly through the hair and sleeping on rollers are the two most common forms of feminine mistreatment. Rollers worn tight for long periods are also responsible for hair loss. Hairdressers and dermatologists note that thinning hair and balding seem to be on the increase among both men and women. Since a majority of people go on secretly worrying about thinning hair without ever visiting a professional, the odds are that the number of people affected by this problem is considerably larger than is generally suspected.

Correction: The idea that the problem will disappear is simply wishful thinking. Without seeking professional help, chances are that more hair will disappear before the problem does. If your hair shows signs of excessive thinning, a visit to your family physician is in order, followed by a visit to a dermatologist. Professional men may be able to trace your hair loss to a recent illness, or possibly to an emotional upset—in which case the lost hair will return normally. Only through bona fide medical experts will you be able to pinpoint the cause and cures for your hair loss.

There is an ancient receipt originating, it is said, in Puerto Rico, which has been handed down by word of mouth for generations. This formula against falling hair calls for a visit to a handcraft shoemaker to collect bits and scrapings of leather shavings. Plenty of water is added to the scrapings as well as a sprig of savory, a handful of cloves, ground flax, leeks, and comfrey. Simmer for five to six hours. The ingredients are left on the hair overnight before being washed out. Unfortunately, although this recipe has survived for many generations, there is no money-back guarantee.

Glover's Mange is a product normally prescribed by veterinarians to correct the mangy hair of cats and dogs. This product has been reputed to be an army technique to counterattack falling hair amongst military personnel. The product is applied to the hair and left on for a minimum half-hour. Reports are that the longer it is left on the head before being washed out, the better. Those who have used it say the cure is just as strong as its aroma.

Redken Laboratories produces P.P.T. "S-77," a special conditioning formula full of wonder-working polypeptides, nature's own proteins. Experimental confirmation demonstrating that amino acid proteins (polypeptides) are actually absorbed by the hair was reported in the *Journal of Cosmetic Society* in July 1959. As a general conditioner, the solution is combed through freshly washed hair and left on for twenty minutes or more before being rinsed out. P.P.T. "S-77" helps to prevent embrittlement, stops breakage, and aids in restoring natural body and elasticity to the hair. This product is available through beauty supply houses and special drugstores; it is very frequently used in professional salons. If your hair shows noticeable signs of thinning, try the formula before you've nothing left to lose.

Pure Silvikrin, an organic hair-food product, manufactured by the Silvikrin Laboratories in England and sold in special drugstores in the United States (Caswell-Massey Co., Ltd., 518 Lexington Ave., New York City), is a valuable aid to combatting thinning hair. The green lotion, massaged into the scalp daily, acts as a catalyst to improve circulation and hair growth. It is not sticky. Good results have been reported by most users who highly praise the benefits of this product.

Without taking dramatic steps, you can do your part in preserving your hair by maintaining a proper diet, getting plenty of rest, keeping cool and calm, and treating your hair with utmost gentleness. It cannot be stated often enough—*never* sleep on rollers. Another tip: keep your hair at one length. According to George Michaels, two-thirds of your hair may fall out if you cut your hair at varying lengths. He claims the body naturally seeks to maintain a state of equilibrium; therefore, if you cut bangs, the back of your hair will do its utmost to break or shed in an effort to balance the front portion of your hair.

Sparse hair can be made to look artificially fuller by wearing it at a medium length, fluffed up. A little assist from a partial hairpiece may help to provide renewed confidence. Steer away from products or individuals claiming to have magical cures for thinning hair. Do not rely solely on artificial means of improvement; rely on the sound advice of your doctor and follow his instructions to the letter.

Baldness

Going, going, gone; baldness is the ultimate in thinning hair. The scalp is either partially barren or totally without hair.

As you will see, there are several theories regarding the cause of baldness.

> Babies haven't any hair,
> Old men's heads are just as bare,
> Between the cradle and the grave
> Lies a haircut and a shave.

This ditty by S. Hoffenstein seems to infer that baldness is simply in the hands of destiny.

"A good man grows gray, but a rascal grows bald," observes a Czech proverb, implying a moral cause for balding. And here's a concept without rhyme or reason: There's one thing about baldness—it's neat.

The poet Ovid summed it up succinctly when he proclaimed, "Ugly is a field without grass, a plant without leaves or a head without hair."

Since the beginning of recorded time, people have been vainly seeking the causes and cures for baldness. Over 5,000 years ago an Egyptian queen reportedly used a concoction of dogs' toes, the hoof of an ass, and date husks in an attempt to restore her hair. The oldest medical text in existence, *The Papyrus Ebers*, prescribes the fat of a lion, a hippo, a crocodile, a serpent, and an ibex.

Cause: Most experts today agree that male baldness normally stems from an inherited disorder which generally appears in early adult life, without necessarily being preceded by either oiliness or dandruff.

Those who hold a naturalist point of view agree that although baldness may be an inherited weakness, the possibility of preventing the condition from occurring or from spreading does exist. In fact, with proper care, it is possible to strengthen the hair and to promote its growth. Naturalists contend that baldness is more often due to a contraction of the blood vessels, which ultimately inhibits proper nourishment from reaching the scalp. Contraction, they say, is usually due to some form of nervous tension, or due to pressure exerted on the blood vessels of the scalp by the continual wearing of tight hats. Lastly is the contention that lack of mineral salts in the diet is a serious contributing factor.

Under no circumstances do naturalists consider baldness to be incurable. What may be thought to be an inherited disorder may only mean that son, like father, has been subject to a poor diet, or has experienced similar nervous frustrations; therefore, the muscles of the neck in both parent and child have become contracted to such a degree that the head is constantly kept at an angle that constricts circulation.

Even when the blood supply to the scalp is efficient, the blood itself may be undernourished. Ample mineral salts and vitamins must be supplied by the food we eat in order to enrich the blood which circulates to the scalp.

The Five Stages of Balding

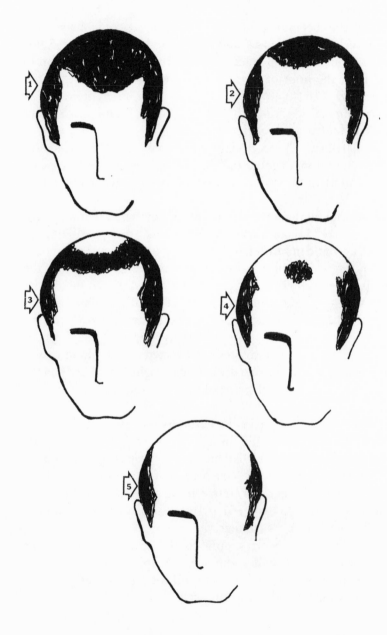

Traction Baldness Caused by a Tightly Pulled Ponytail

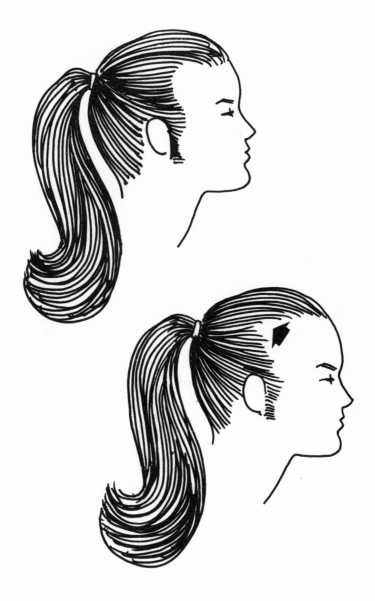

Correction: Natural cures for baldness naturally include dietary improvements. Artificial sun-ray treatments are also recommended, although the natural rays of the sun are even more beneficial. Sun treatments should be taken three times a week, and immediate results should not be expected. Noticeable hair growth doesn't occur overnight, even on the healthiest of heads. Over an extended period, sun stimulation, air stimulation, and relaxation techniques will help bring about improvements. Immediate attention should be paid to thinning or falling hair. If baldness is allowed to progress, the hair follicles may close up and lose their functioning power completely. In this event, hair growth will not take place.

Without effort, there will be no gains. Naturalists claim that one of the best ways to relax the body, which includes the scalp, is to lie lightly clad on the grass, weather permitting, so that the magnetism of the earth is taken into the body, thereby recharging it with energy. Walking barefoot on the grass also helps to release nervous tensions. Neck exercises such as rolling the head in a circular movement from left to right and right to left, should be practiced daily. Massaging the scalp with the fingertips is also a daily must. To stimulate the scalp, it is recommended that women comb their hair with a comb that has been dipped into cold water.

Women, except when affected by disease, do not normally experience any noticeable degree of baldness; nor is childbirth a cause of female baldness as it is sometimes claimed. The hormonal imbalance and physical stress of pregnancy may, in some women, force hair into a premature resting phase, so that hair loss becomes apparent. This is, however, only a temporary condition.

There are those who do not go along with a naturalistic point of view and simply say that baldness cannot be cured by local remedies or by oral means, such as foods, pills, or potions; that the one cure for baldness is a toupee or wig.

If baldness is truly not a hereditary condition, there seems to be a chance for regrowth of hair, so long as the hair follicles are not dead. Where there is life, there is hope, when and if proper effort is extended.

10.
Shampooing

The products best for your hair are dependent on your hair's characteristics. Therefore, by becoming better acquainted with your hair, and determining its type—oily, dry, fine, coarse, too thick, or too thin—the selection of a shampoo is made easier.

Advice from the experts regarding shampoo products often seems perplexing. Points of view differ radically; however, in the final analysis, the alternate positions taken will help you reach your own decision as to which shampoo is most suitable for your own needs.

Herbal Shampoos

Ivan Popov, a Yugoslavian biochemist known for his work in rejuvenation, positively asserts that there is no real difference between the product you normally wash your hair with and that with which you wash your car. Popov believes they are expensive and has a little perfume and natural essences. According to Popov, every shampoo on the market is a bad shampoo. As a biochemist, his answer to this problem is to use a biological detergent instead—which he admits is expensive. Egg shampoos are good, says Popov, except when soap or chemical detergents are used in the shampoo.

Another point of view comes from professional hairdresser Stephen Ball, who operates his Organic Hair Care Center in Mill Valley, California. The only products which he uses and endorses are organic and entirely natural products. With an organic shampoo you have to soap more often, but, says Mr. Ball, hair becomes wildly, wonderfully clean. The house shampoo at the Organic Hair Care Center is a blend of jaborandi, rosemary, southernwood, lemon oil, and camomile in a castile base. Although herbs for beautifying the hair have been used for centuries, they are finding new meaning and importance in our own time.

The problem with herb-shampoo recipes is often one of locating the correct ingredients; however, with any amount of perseverance, you can create your own organic shampoo by following the instructions listed below.

Normal Hair

Fill a sauce pan with water and bring to a boil. Add a heaping teaspoonful of each of the following herbs: nettle, sage, mainden hair, southernwood and peace leaves. Allow to simmer for 15 to 20 minutes. Strain and add shavings of castile soap while the liquid is still warm enough to dissolve. As an alternate recipe, place 1 cup of camomile blossoms in 1 quart of water. Simmer for 10 minutes. Strain and add 1 ounce of castile soap shavings.

Oily Hair—Blond

To absorb excess oil, lightly sprinkle the hair thoroughly with powdered orris. After 5 to 10 minutes, brush out powder. When

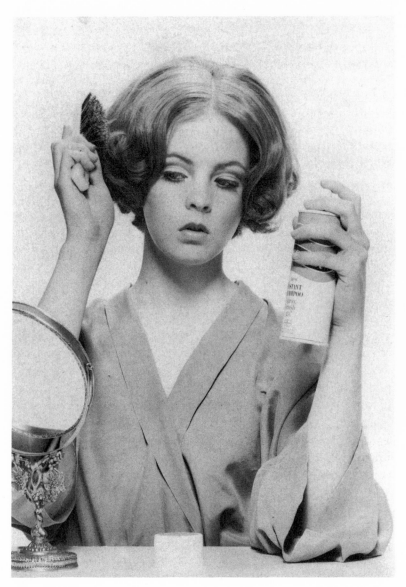

Oil and dirt take a fast powder between regular shampoos with use of a dry shampoo. Courtesy of Clairol Inc.

applied in the evening, it may be left on the entire night and brushed out in the morning.

Oily Hair—Brunette

For black or brown, lifeless hair, boil 1/4 ounce of southernwood, 1/4 ounce of rosemary, 1/4 ounce of rosemary, and 1/4 ounce of quassia chips in enough water to make a wash. Allow to simmer for 10 minutes. Strain and add castile soap shavings. When cool, shampoo with this solution.

Most of us must avail ourselves of those shampoo products which can be purchased over the counter. Amongst those available are many low- or non-detergent shampoos which do the job they were intended for. Breck Shampoo, and Helen Curtis Windsor—available only in beauty supply stores—are among the very best. Neutrogena offers sound nondetergent help with its hypoallergenic cool green solid bar of shampoo; you rub it right on your hair. The Wella Hair Care Company has come up with a new herbal conditioning shampoo which contains extracts of nine nourishing herbs, including nettle which stimulates growth and shine. Ozone's Conditioning Shampoo with herbs and balsam is another newcomer to make hair bloom with health and sparkle. Redken Amino Pon K11 Shampoo features a protein base and an acid balance. Alberto VO5 prepares a good egg shampoo. Head and Shoulders and Enden, used on the average of twice a week work well for sufferers of normal dandruff. Selsun, available only by prescription, is also an excellent dandruff shampoo. For limp hair there are protein shampoos such as Breck's Protein Texturizing Shampoo. In all cases, a good shampoo is not all detergent, has a balance of cleansing and conditioning agents, and works efficiently to keep hair fresh. No matter what the condition of your hair, everyone should be able to find a shampoo that does the job to complete satisfaction.

Choosing a Shampoo

How do you begin selecting the best shampoo for you? Normally, just by experimenting. Manufacturers lend a helping hand by specifying oily hair, dry hair, normal hair, dyed or tinted hair, etcetera, etcetera. If dandruff is your problem, there are many mild dandruff shampoos available from which to choose. For chronic dandruff cases, ask your pharmacist or doctor for his recommendation. For normal or dry hair, a protein shampoo is helpful as it removes less natural oils. Although there are differing opinions on how proteins are assimilated by the hair, it is known that protein shampoos adhere to the hair and do add extra body and smoothness. Egg shampoos contain protein and are especially beneficial for both limp and thin hair. If you're skeptical about the store-bought kind, you can make your own by following this recipe.

Egg Shampoo

Rinse hair and towel dry. Separate three eggs. Whip whites till frothy. Add a tablespoon of water to yolks, and stir to a creamy consistency. Combine whites and yolks. Massage 1/2 mixture into hair. Rinse; then apply remaining egg mixture. Rinse thoroughly with lukewarm water, and dry. Watch your dull hair take on new shine.

For very fine, dry, or damaged hair there are baby shampoos, which can be used by children and adults with equal success. Lemon shampoos leave no dulling film, have a mild lightening effect on blond hair, and are beneficial for all hair tones, except dry hair. White Rain Shampoo with lemon is especially nice for oily hair. Another helpful pointer, if you live in a soft-water community, a castile-based shampoo will give you better results. If the water in your area is hard, a detergent type will do a better job.

Try various shampoos according to your hair type until you find one that gives your hair the feel and texture you want. Finding the right shampoo is extremely important, as the wrong shampoo can leave your hair dull and faded looking. Experiment with baby shampoo, plain castile shampoo, egg shampoo, herbal shampoo, organic shampoo, creme and conditioning shampoos—one is right for your hair. If you can't make up your mind where to begin, start by following these clues.

Normal hair: Any bland high grade castile-type shampoo labeled "For Normal Hair."

Dry hair: A conditioning-formula shampoo with lanolin, or any shampoo labeled "For Dry Hair."

Unmanageable hair: A creme shampoo is recommended unless hair is tinted, dyed, or bleached. In this case, a castile shampoo formulated for color-processed hair will be more effective.

Thick hair: A creme shampoo is best.

Dandruff—oily scalp: Frequent shampooing with a bland shampoo is recommended.

Dandruff—dry scalp: Use a mild shampoo, don't wash too frequently, and follow the recommendations offered for dry hair.

Oily hair: Lather frequently with a bland shampoo or one formulated specificatlly "For Oily Hair."

Fine or limp hair: A regular mild castile shampoo or a protein shampoo will help, as will frequent shampooing.

Tinted hair: Use a mild castile shampoo, one specially formulated for tinted or bleached hair.

Gray hair: A shampoo "For Gray Hair" will wash away dingy yellow and enliven color.

Before you shampoo, take the time to give your hair a good brushing to loosen it of any surface dirt and to get out tangles which tend to turn into knots once the hair is wet. A few minutes massaging your scalp are minutes well spent.

There are well-known professionals who believe in devoting up to one entire hour preparing the scalp before proceeding to the ritual of shampooing. Preshampoo treatment begins with a neck and shoulder massage to relax tensions. Thereafter, the massage progresses to the scalp, starting at the point right above the ears and at the base of the skull, to help encourage proper blood circulation. After virgorous massaging, a heat cap may be used to open pores so as to further prepare the scalp for the shampoo cleansing which is to follow.

This may all seem extreme to you, but if you have the time, try it. The results are really very beneficial. In any case, spend at least 5 minutes brushing and massaging to achieve a loose, supple scalp. Only then are you truly ready to start your shampoo.

Next, douse your hair with plenty of warm water—not hot. Ideally, science tells us, distilled water is best. Rain water does nicely. Tap water suffices. In any case, apply shampoo generously and massage with your fingertips. Always work from the scalp outward to the ends of the hair. To help your scalp remain loose, shampoo in an upside-down position. (If you keep your elbows above your head, the scalp tenses up automatically. Just try it for yourself and see.) For long hair, shampoo *with* the length of the hair, not across it. Use long strokes, preferably while under the shower. Creep up under hair and let your fingers go to work on the scalp in an up-and-down motion. Short hairs have more latitude and can be worked up, down, in zigzags or circles because the hair isn't long enough to become tangled.

Lots of lathering and lots of suds are not necessary during your first sudsing session; this bout is meant to rid the scalp and hair of surface soil. It is in the second sudsing that you really get down to nitty-gritty basics. Rinse well and repeat.

On the second round, lather well and massage and massage and massage. The better the massage, the looser and cleaner your scalp will be. Use not-too-hot water. Cool it. Your head gets just as clean and will feel better if you keep the temperature down. If you have an adjustable shower nozzle which allows for a fine strong spray, your final rinse will be easier.

Investing in a home spray hose which can be attached to the sink or shower faucet is well worthwhile. Whether with or without a hose attachment, rinse, rinse, and rerinse. *Note:* Warm water dissolves shampoo alkali better than cold water, but the idea that cold water hardens the hair is a fantasy. Whether washing or rinsing, water should be kept warm to cool, never steaming hot nor icy cold.

Hair may be difficult to handle after washing, in which case a creme rinse may be the answer. There are creme rinses especially for blonde hair, for coarse-textured stiff hair that tangles, for normal hair that needs more control. There's even a creme rinse for fine, flyaway hair that tangles. They're all part of the Breck line of hair-care products.

After the final rinsing, wrap up your head in a terry towel, turban style, and blot up all the excess water. Do not wring your hair. Wet hair stretches and is therefore more susceptible to breakage. Hair should be dried immediately. Lengthy drying results in the slow evaporation of water, thereby causing loss of moisture content in the hair, leaving it dry and brittle. Too much heat also overevaporates moisture content. When using a dryer, play it cool. Never brush wet hair. Use a wide-tooth comb, gently, so that your hair is free of any tangles. Incidentally, be sure to keep your combs and brushes clean. They should be washed just as often as you wash your hair.

Which brings up another question. Can hair be washed too often? The answer is no—unless you have been tampering with cemicals, bleaches, or straightening products, or are using a shampoo which is too harsh for your head. Experts feel that it is better to wash more often and even less thoroughly than to wash less often. The general rule is shampoo as often as you can do so comfortably. If you wash your hair a lot, one good sudsing is probably all you need. Shampooing less than once a week indicates a poor hair-care program. Oily hair should be washed at minimum twice a week. In fact, Dr. Norman Orentreich, New York dermatologist, recommends lots of shampooing, twice a week minimum or every day for those with hair which has not been damaged by chemicals. Keeping the scalp clean helps prevent dandruff, infection, and loss of hair. Living in a sooty atmosphere or visiting a sandy beach area can mean washing hair every day in order to keep it in top-notch condition.

Oil and dirt take a fast powder between regular shampoos with use of a dry shampoo. These are basically powder formulas that you shake or spray right onto the hair. Popular brands available at drugstore counters everywhere include Breck Fresh Hair, Minipoo, Pssssst Instant Shampoo, and Mini Mist. All you do is apply generously, wait a few minutes to allow the powder to absorb oil and dust particles, then brush your hair until the powder is gone.

Surprisingly enough, some people with gorgeous hair never shampoo it. That is to say, they never get their hair wet and sudsy. Instead, they rub oatmeal into the scalp and hair and energetically comb it through the strands to remove soil. In India, clean potter's clay or soapnut powder is often used to keep hair looking shiny and clean.

Here is an exotic dry shampoo you can make yourself. Mix and sieve 1/2 pound of powdered orris root together with 2-3/4 drams each of dried bergamot rind and cassis flowers, plus 1/2 dram of coarsely ground cloves. Powder the hair with the mixture and leave on all night. In the morning brush it out.

Dry shampoos offer the advantage of being quick pick-me-ups, without upsetting hair styling. Although they are real lifesavers for last-minute occasions, they are not meant to replace regular shampooing by any means.

Keeping hair scrupulously clean is not just another cliché. It's an absolute necessity to achieve or maintain a healthy scalp and fantastic-looking hair.

11.
Hair Conditioners

Making peace with your hair calls for finding the proper solution for its present unhappy state. The only time to get a really good feel for the situation is while the hair is wet. Start getting the problem in hand by shampooing and then rinsing. If the strands feel sticky or limp or if the hair combs out in large clumps or if you can't pull the comb through your hair, don't fight. Surrender conditionally. There are teams of rescuers at your command in the form of conditioning agents.

No matter what problem exists, the function of virtually every conditioning products is to replace the oils and proteins both you and nature have taken out of your hair. Regardless of your hair's present state, a conditioner will help it look and behave better. Conditioners bind moisture into the hair, to keep it from feeling coarse and brittle, to keep it from breaking, and to let it shine. Remember, too, that conditioners are not limited to use solely by women; they are for men, too, and should be used by anyone who wants to improve the feel and texture of his or her hair.

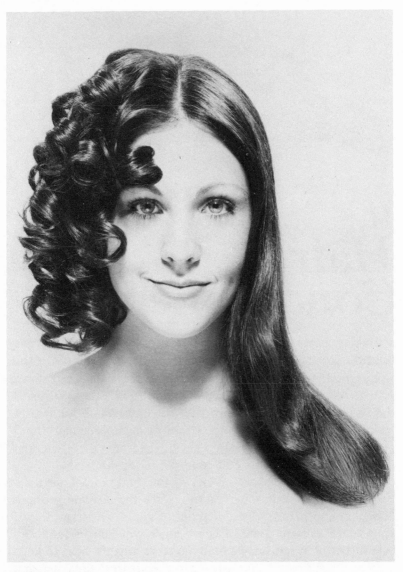

Making peace with your hair calls for finding the proper solution to its present unhappy state. Courtesy of Clairol Inc.

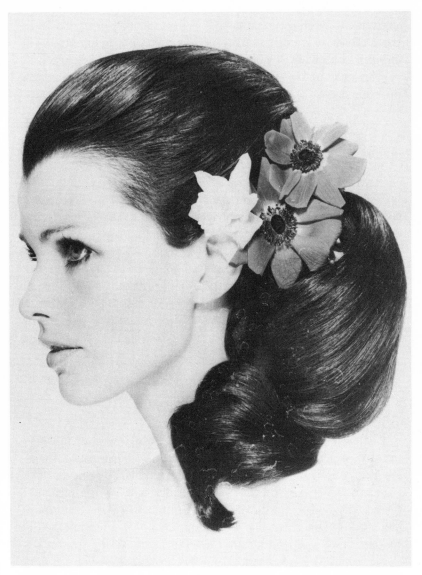

Simple off-the-face styles will keep you looking fresh and appealing all summer long. Courtesy of Clairol Inc.

How do you know which conditioner works best? The right one depends on how you have been treating your hair, its subsequent condition, and the season of the year. Basically there are two types of conditioners (which does help narrow the choices somewhat). You can select either a deep-penetrating conditioner or an instant conditioner, depending upon the problem.

Deep-Penetrating Conditioners

For real correction of damaged hair—hair that shows breakage, split ends, brittleness or unmanageability caused by overspraying, teasing, bleaching, untimely straightening, or permanenting—deep-penetrating conditioners are the answer. This type is applied to the hair and scalp and remains there for approximately twenty minutes before being rinsed out. A small sampling of popular brand names includes these deep conditioners—Breck Satin, Revlon's Flex, Clairol's Condition, L'Oreal's Ineral, and Wella Kolestral.

Instant Conditioners

For added fullness, body, smoothness of line and improved texture—especially for thin, fine, limp, and hard-to-hold hair—instant conditioners do the job. These magical potions often come in little vials or tubes specifically labeled for bleached, tinted, dry, oily, or normal hair. Contents are applied to the hair and remain there one to five minutes or until the next time you shampoo, depending on what the manufacturer prescribes. Some are rinsed away and some are not. Instant conditioning products include the Treatment de Pantene; Clairol's Kindness; as well as Clairol's Great Body for very straight hair, and Clairol's Long & Silk Conditioning Lotion for long hair;

L'Oreal's Suffrage; Wella Gentle Care; Bio-Kur; Get Set Swinging Body; and—for soft holding power and silkiness for coarse or wiry hair—Breck Basic's Silk 'N Hold gives top-notch first aid. The most popular rinse-out instant conditioner is Balsam. This name is marketed by many major hair-care companies including Wella, Carrol Richards, Revlon, and Ozone.

For ridding hair of tangles, and adding sheen and manageability, creme rinses come to the rescue by reducing hair's static electricity so that it behaves properly instead of retaliating. Creme rinses work like deep-penetrating conditioners and are always rinsed out. Because they are less powerful than twenty-minute deep-conditioning products, they are not intended for repairing seriously damaged hair.

Conditioning ingredients are now contained in practically all modern hair-care products, even shampoos. Protein, a restorative, is often a conditioning additive on the principle that hair is pure protein in the first place. Protein additives propose to replenish and reinforce fading protein by either penetrating or clinging to the hair shafts.

Although conditioners are recommended by all professionals, some suggest using half doses, which they say do equally well without leaving any sticky coating on the hair. Rudel offers this timely word of caution—daily conditioning in the form of rinses to soften hair and hardeners for setting, put hair through changes which, if kept up night after night and day after day, will lead to hair breakage rather than hair improvement. Overconditioning is no better than underconditioning.

Just how much is too much and how much is too little? The proper proportion is a simple, faithful, once-a-week treatment. If the hair is badly damaged, a heating cap or hot towel wrapped securely around the head will help to intensify the benefits of a weekly conditioning session.

Regardless of which conditioner you select, the method of application always follows the same pattern. To be 100 percent effective all conditioners must be applied to damp, freshly washed hair. The conditioning solution must be evenly distributed through all of the hair strands, preferably combed through and left for the time period specified by the maker. Rinsing may or may not be required. Be sure to check directions carefully.

Season, too, will influence your conditioning program. During the winter, hair is subject to more abuse because of more drastic temperature changes. It may be zero degrees on the outside and seventy-five on the inside. As a result, hair is in a constant state of flux, shrinking and expanding. Steam heat, drying winds, and air pollution are added wintertime hazards. Most often, because of freezing temperatures, winter hair is in a shrunken state. A hair conditioner such as Wella's Balsam treatment will help to normalize winterized hair in just sixty seconds.

During summer months the problem reverses itself. When the heat is on, hair molecules move apart, increasing the diameter of the hair shaft. Now a twenty-minute deep-conditioning treatment is needed because of larger spaces between molecules and its deeper penetrating action. Revlon's Flex and Tame's Creme-Rinse Conditioner help to keep summer hair manageable. For added protection from summertime hair hazards, take heed. If you abhor bathing caps, before plunging into the salty brine remember to rub a deep-conditioning creme lightly over your hair just before you dive in. This will help protect your hair against the drying effects of both salt and sun. Also remember to pool your interests. If you swim in a chlorinated pool, try using an undiluted creme rinse on your locks before jumping in. Breck's pink creme rinse dilutes the chances of chemical harm to hair and makes the pool water softer for you and the other swimmers.

The best time to head full swing into a program of hair conditioning is during the spring. It is the ideal time to repair winter hair damage and to prepare against possible damage from the sun's brilliant summer rays. If you've missed out on a spring conditioning, start; don't wait until next season. A hair conditioning program should be a year-round ritual with but only minor variations due to seasonal changes.

The Miracle of Conditioning as Seen through a Microscope

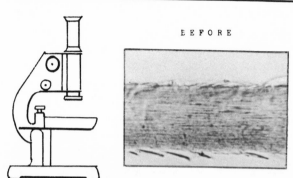

BEFORE

After: The miracle of conditioning is demonstrated. When the strand is treated with proteins, a healthy state returns. Scales of the cuticle appear flat and smooth, thereby restoring proper protection to the cortex. The medulla reappears, although intermittently. Conclusion: A conditioning program with the right ingredients helps maintain and restore hair's elasticity, strength and proper moisture content.

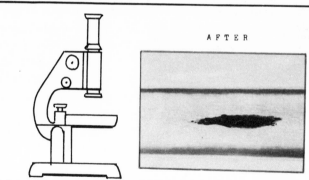

AFTER

Before: The above is a damaged human hair magnified over 100 times. Cuticle scales show breakage and are literally worn away. Possible causes for this condition may be natural or chemical—too much sun, or air oxidation, drying winds, hard or salt water, harsh bleaches, tints, permanent waves or the wrong shampoo. As is characteristic of ill health, the medulla does not appear at all.

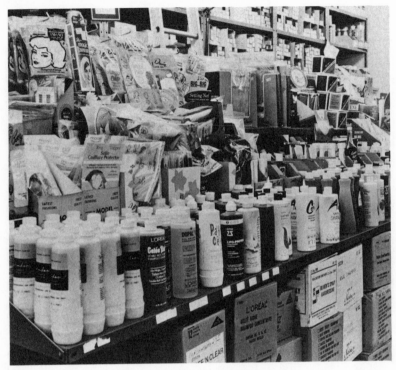

The abundance of hair products on the market today offers a solution for every problem, as demonstrated at Ray Beauty Supply Co., N.Y.C.

Summer, winter, spring, or fall, the number of conditioners available for ailing locks is abundant. No matter how the products are packaged—whether a jar, tube, or vial—you will be able to find a product which will help make your hair more supple, more lustrous and more manageable. In addition to conditioners meant solely for repairing hair ills, shampoos, rinses, and hairdressing cremes are also chock-full of conditioning ingredients to offer hair dual benefits. It should be noted that rinses containing lemon, beer, or vinegar—although uniquely beneficial to fine and chemically treated hair—are not, in a true sense, conditioners. When used after shampooing or conditioning treatments, these rinses act to neutralize residual alkali or cleansing and beautifying agents; thus hair is left feeling silky and more manageable simply because the rinsing action is more thorough. Products such as Brill Creme ("a little dab'll do ya"), Helene Curtis's Suave, Long Aid K7, Avon's Hair Sheen Dressing, or Afro Sheen do legitimately perform dual functions. Each doubles as a groomer and a daily conditioner to combat dull, dry, or brittle hair.

For dry hair, hot oil treatments act as a beneficial supplement to regular conditioning treatments. Unlike regular conditioning products which are rinsed out, hot oil conditioners must be shampooed out prior to the final rinse. Dousing your scalp and hair with vegetable or baby oil may be a bit messy but if your hair is extra parched and dry, the treatment is well worth the extra fuss.

Beneficial homemade organic conditioners are also a possibility. You can go mildly organic, for example, with mayonnaise. Why not? After all, mayonnaise contains nature's own healthful, glorifying hair ingredients: eggs, oil, and vinegar. Spread two heaping teasponfuls through your hair. Wait twenty minutes, rinse thoroughly, and behold—you have hair that shines with health!

Flower power also offers naturally unique healing powers. Besides flowers, both herbs and essences have been used for centuries by nature lovers as a hair aid: eucalyptus for circulation; nasturtium and boxwood to fortify roots; henna to beautifully sheathe hair; thyme and rosemary to add essential oils; and cress to cut oil. Although ever popular in Europe, the importance of flowers, herbs, and essences is just beginning to bloom in our own society.

The very latest witness to this fact is the introduction of Estee Lauder's Azuree collection of hair treatments, all richly endowed with herbs, vegetable oils, and natural proteins to make hair supple, glossy, and vibrantly alive: Azuree Single-Application Natural Shampoo; Azuree Natural Rinse—for dry, normal, and oily hair—to help smooth and condition flyaway locks; Azuree Naturally Enriched Setting Spray, to make fine hair look fuller, thick hair more natural; and Azuree Herbal

Pack Condition and Nourisher, a rich treatment that coats each stand with health and is especially helpful for reconditioning dull, dry, sun-damaged, or chemically treated hair. From Avanene comes more natural help in the form of avocado-based products brimming with proteins and vitamins including Avanene Organic Avocado Shampoo and Hair Conditioner. On the basis that malt is a hair marvel, Aramis has introduced malt-enriched products for men—shampoo and conditioners—to help hair feel and look thicker. You can return to nature by paying a visit to one of the fine department stores in your area or, theoretically, by brewing your own conditioner, based on one of the following formulas:

Nettle Rinse

Adds body to fine hair. Place one handful of nettles in one quart of water. Strain and apply liquid to the hair. Whether you do or do not set your hair, when dried and combed, hair will be fluffy and full. By rubbing a few drops of rosemary oil into the hair, you will gain added sheen.

Camomile Rinse

Delicately lightens locks. Steep these daisylike dried flowers for approximately 10 minutes in boiling water, 2 tablespoons to a quart. Strain contents. When cool, pour the solution through the hair. When hair reaches the desired shade, rinse out.

Nettle Conditioner

Put a handful of nettles into one quart of water and boil for 2 hours. When cool, strain and bottle, apply the solution to the scalp every other night. This conditioner must be prepared fresh every three to four days so as to retain its softening and glossening powers.

Parsnip Root Conditioner

Place one chopped parsnip root and 1/2 teaspoon of parsnip seeds in 1/4 cup of olive oil. Boil for 5 minutes, strain, and rub liquid into scalp and hair. This conditioning lotion adds gloss and helps deter hair loss.

Cherry Bark Conditioner

Peel the bark from a wild cherrywood tree, boil it over a low flame for 20 minutes. Strain and cool. This solution is used as a wash and is considered as an excellent hair conditioner. Good results are said to be seen in as little as one month's time.

Regardless of the product you select to use, after two months of faithful weekly conditioning treatments, your hair will be easier to handle, better looking, and in far superior condition. Don't be surprised if a friend tells you how great your hair looks—it's your reward for maintaining a faithful conditioning campaign.

12.
Hair Sprays

Over 300 million cans of hair spray are sold yearly in the United States, which clearly indicates that aerosol hair sprays are here to stay. There are poof formulas for hard-to-hold hair, for fine hair, for bleached hair, for normal hair; sprays to add shine, sprays specifically for wigs and falls; and now sprays specifically designed for the male market. Many sprays feature built-in conditioners, shiners, or protein ingredients. In any spray, the chief ingredient used to keep hair in place is a resin called polyvinyl pyrrolidone. This holding resin is contained within an alcohol base to which Freon is added to jet the spray from the can. All three ingredients are shampoo soluble and can be washed out. Today very few sprays contain harmful lacquers.

Modern hair sprays are a big boon to keeping hair looking neat. Today's sprays are usually nonstiffening, nonsticky, and leave little or no spray buildup on the hair—nor do they alter hair color. They merely provide natural-looking staying power without dulling the hair.

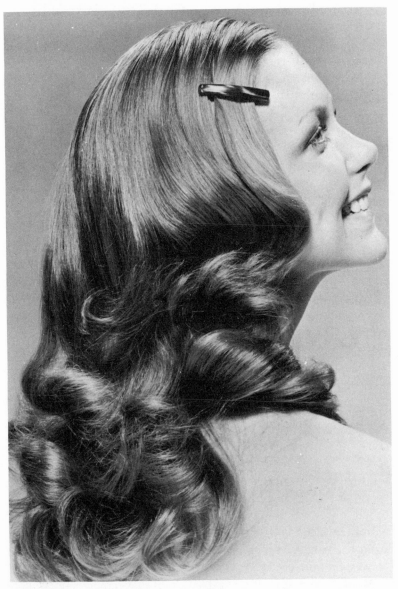

Hair can be beautiful only when it looks and feels like hair.
Courtesy of Clairol Inc.

Historically, women have used hair-control preparations for centuries, generally in the form of creams, pomades, or hardeners. Even Cleopatra made use of some form of hardener to keep her hair free of ripples, and Marie Antoinette's curly coiffures, too, were held together by some form of artificial hardener, as were the sculptured curls of Japanese geisha girls.

Modern setting gels, lotions, and pomades have not changed radically from their ancient formulas and still serve the very same purpose. With or without proteins, Dep Styling Gel, Get Set gel or lotion, Mennen's Protein Hair Groomer, and Posner's Pomatex are used to keep hair in place, just as yesterday's creams, hardeners, and pomades did. The only new innovation in staying power since the reign of Cleopatra is our aerosol hair sprays.

With over one hundred well-known and private labels, or chain-brand labels, women have a giant selection of names from which to choose. Aquanet and Just Wonderful are the two leading brands. The combined sales of these two alone in 1970 totaled almost fifty-million dollars.

The number-one best seller among men's hair sprays is Faberge's Brut. Before Brut made the scene, most men unobtrusively lifted the little lady's can of spray. Now that longer hair is here, a variety of new hair sprays for men have sprung up. Among the new entries are such names as General, Command, Consort, Dep Men's Hair Spray, Vitalis Dry Control, and Hair Mist for Men. Obviously, men are also succumbing to the powerful grip of today's holding sprays.

With such a variety of sprays on the market, how do you find the one that is best for you? The answer: Simply by trying several brands which feature different purposes and ingredients (hard-to-hold, normal, nonallergenic, protein, lanolin, etc.), until you find one that doesn't leave your hair looking lacquered, glued-together or dull. There are a number of good sprays on the market. When possible, try experimenting with small cans of spray until you find one that is exactly right for your hair.

Not everybody uses or needs a hair spray. If your hair falls and stays in place naturally, don't bother adding unnecessary spray chemicals. There are lots of women, and men too, who feel their hair is incomplete unless they add spray. It's a kind of security blanket against the natural forces of wind and rain which can easily make a mess out of well-styled hair. Today, 16 to 22 year olds rarely use sprays because the longer, casual hair styles don't require a spray. When shorter, curlier styles become the rage, those who don't need a spray now may need one later.

Sprays should never be used as a substitute for setting lotions or permanent waving; they are meant to hold hair in place and should be used sparingly to achieve a natural look, not a rigid look. Excessive spraying means you must shampoo sooner. When spraying, hold the can at least ten inches away from your head. Always spray from a side or a back angle. Never spray towards either the face or eyes. There are cases where women have suffered nose or eye irritations from spray. This may be the result of using the wrong spray or spraying incorrectly. If irritations occur every time you spray, stop spraying. To date, nobody has ever died from an overdose of hair spray, but that's no license to overspray, by any means. Spraying should be done in moderation and with the correct product. A little spray is all you need to give your hair added body. Once hair is soaked with spray, it looks and feels sticky. Instead of adding to your appeal, overspraying will make you a hard-looking, sticky mess. Remember, no one longs to run their fingers through shellacked locks.

Some quick hair spray tips (but don't overdo any one of them): For a very quick set, set hair in pins or rollers, spray each curl and allow to dry. After final combing and arranging, spray once again lightly. If a curl or two begins to droop and you're out of hair spray, use an atomizer filled with a fast-evaporating cologne as a substitute. For more control, use a light amount of nondrying, low-moisture spray after brushing hair. The best advice—never, never overspray!

Some professionals insist that sprays should be washed out as soon as possible, preferably before going to bed at night. Others say hair spray should be brushed out at the end of each day. What is important is that you never allow hair spray to build up, as this causes dry hair. Furthermore, too much spray inhibits your scalp from breathing properly. If hair spray is allowed to remain on the scalp for excessive periods, scalp infections may occur as a result of chemical reactions. Unlike the sprays of yesteryear, most of today's hair sprays are water soluble and can be easily washed out—and should be for safety's sake. The most important lessons are don't overspray, and don't allow spray to build up. Hair can be beautiful only when it looks and feels like hair.

13.
Hair and Scalp Exercises

Brushing

Stimulation is a big word which means exercise for both hair and scalp. Brushing is the biggest and best exerciser. Nothing gleams better than well-brushed hair and nothing brushes it better than a standard hairbrush.

Brushing may seem like an old-fashioned idea, but it really helps to keep hair vitally clean, healthy, and in the best of shape. With the help of a hairbrush, surface dust and dirt lift away, the scalp is stimulated to function normally, and hair is kept manageable and tangle-free. On top of everything else, the power of a hairbrush is one of the greatest conditioners available. Daily brushing prevents excess oil from collecting and flaking on the scalp while helping to lubricate the hair by spreading natural oils from roots to ends. That's how nice, shiny, polished hair happens.

When it comes to selecting a hairbrush, it doesn't pay to economize. Good ones last longer and are well worth having.

Should you buy a nylon or a natural-bristled brush? If they have the right qualities, why not buy one of each—natural bristles for daily use, to remove dust, to distribute oils, and to check static electricity; and nylon bristles for before shampooing sessions, to loosen dirt and to stimulate the scalp. In both instances, the brush handle must feel comfortable and the brush must be free of split bristles. When selecting a nylon brush, run your fingertips over the bristles to make sure they are rounded and not scratchy. If possible, use a magnifying glass to check the ends of the bristles.

Natural bristles have a tendency to split more quickly than nylon. On the other hand, natural bristles are more flexible and thus are less apt to break any weakened hairs. No matter what, avoid rubber-based brushes. They feed electricity in towards the hair and scalp and weaken the hair.

A good brush ranges in price anywhere from $5 to $30. Styling brushes are smaller, cost a little less, but their general qualifications remain the same. (These miniature brushes are specifically designed for hair-styling purposes, not for stimulation.)

Your hairbrush should be limited to use on dry hair only. Although it's a fact that healthy hair is stronger than steel in that it can expand 1/8 to 1/6 of its full length before it snaps or breaks, wet hair stretches beyond these limits and, therefore, snaps and breaks off more quickly—especially when it is being bristled into shape by a brush.

More bristly news—if you are not accustomed to one-hundred brush strokes a day, don't go overboard the first time around. Start out with twenty strokes the first day and add ten strokes each day thereafter until you finally reach a full hundred strokes. Launching into a high-geared brushing campaign without proper build-up is bound to leave your scalp and arms feeling sore. Ultimately two-hundred or three-hundred strokes a day are fine, and two or three minutes is all the time it takes.

The best time to brush is the first thing in the morning, while circulation is at its greatest. Brush in an upside-down position with your head between your knees. When brushing hair before bedtime, follow the same procedure—bend over and let the blood flow to your scalp. Pull the brush firmly and evenly from the base of the roots to the ends of your hair. Wind up your brushing sessions by straightening up, sectioning your hair, and brushing section by section, until it is all back in place. By doing this you will be giving your hair added fullness without any harmful teasing.

If you're too tired to stand up, lie down. Dangle your head over the end of the bed and brush. When hair is badly tangled, begin brushing at the ends first, working your way up the hair strands to the scalp. By following this course you will be less likely to yank out hairs. As soon as the snarls have disappeared, revert to long, sweeping strokes from scalp to hair ends.

By the way, don't wear nylon or synthetic apparel while brushing; these materials increase static electricity. If you can't get out of your nylon shirt or blouse, be sure you are either wearing sneakers or standing on a rubber mat. This will get rid of the static for you. Avoid tight belts, bras, or collars, which tend to curtail circulation.

Brushing Tips

Dry hair naturally needs extra brushing to spread scalp oils. Try placing several dabs of a lubricating conditioner in the palm of your hand, then running your palm over the bristles of your brush. This allows your hairbrush to distribute extra lubrication to both scalp and locks as you brush.

Oily hair requires superbrushing to prevent oil from collecting and flaking on the scalp. Excess oils can be removed from the hair by taping a piece of muslin to your hair brush to absorb oil while you brush.

Fine or damaged hair needs a soft-bristle brush. Natural bristles are best for damaged hair.

Thin or damaged hair or a *tender scalp condition* require special kindness. Start off with 10 to 20 brush strokes a day, just enough to remove any dead hairs and promote better circulation. Don't yank or pull hair.

Wiry or coarse hair must also be treated gently. Don't yank or pull or you will defeat your purpose. This type of hair needs a hairbrush with extra-long bristles and lots of faithful brushing.

Normal hair requires faithful daily brushing to keep it ever shining and healthy.

Massage

Massage is another form of stimulation recommended because of its healthy benefits to hair and scalp. Like brushing, massaging stimulates oil glands so that hair roots receive proper lubrication and oils are distributed through the hair to keep it glossy and bright. Massaging also aids in increasing circulation in the scalp. It leaves a good tingling feeling that seems to flow right down to the tip of your toes. Massage puts medication in and takes soil and dust away.

Some hair specialists operate on the premise that massaging increases the growth of hair. Whether this is so remains questionable. Although constant manipulation of the hair through massaging can cause hair to become coarser and longer, almost in the same way that constant rubbing of the skin can cause a callous to grow, the main benefit of massaging is to keep the scalp healthy and alive, not to add new hair growth. Massaging does not increase the number of hairs, but it may fatten up those you already have. (Note that the average allotment of hair follicles per head is established during the fourth fetal month, and is usually about 100,000.)

Gentle massages of the scalp for five minutes, twice a day, will do a good part of duplicating the work that brushing does and will enhance your brushing efforts. If hair is dry or normal, massage just as often as time allows; once a day should be the minimum. You can easily massage while watching TV, soaking in the bathtub, or when reading—just prop up your book. Only if

Exercises to Improve Scalp Circulation

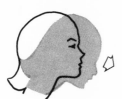

DROP HEAD FORWARD.
RETURN TO UPRIGHT
POSITION. REPEAT 5 TIMES.

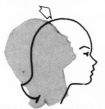

DROP HEAD BACKWARDS.
RETURN TO UPRIGHT
POSITION. REPEAT 5 TIMES.

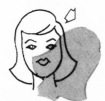

TILT HEAD TO EXTREME LEFT.
RETURN TO UPRIGHT
POSITION. REPEAT 5 TIMES.

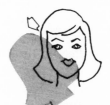

TILT HEAD TO EXTREME RIGHT.
RETURN TO UPRIGHT
POSITION. REPEAT 5 TIMES.

TURN HEAD TO EXTREME LEFT.
RETURN TO ORIGINAL
POSITION. REPEAT 5 TIMES.

TURN HEAD TO EXTREME RIGHT.
RETURN TO ORIGINAL
POSITION. REPEAT 5 TIMES.

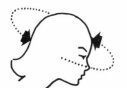

DROP HEAD FORWARD.
ROTATE IT SLOWLY
TO THE LEFT 5 TIMES.

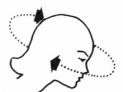

DROP HEAD FORWARD.
ROTATE IT SLOWLY
TO THE RIGHT 5 TIMES.

hair is oily are you allowed to confine your massages to a once-a-week schedule before shampooing.

Get into the swing of helping scalp circulation even more by doing a few basic head exercises. Try this as a starter. Drop your head forward as far as it will go. Raise it upright again. Repeat five times. Next, drop your head back as far as it will go. Raise it upright again. Repeat five times. Swing your head left, center, right. Rotate it five times from left to right, then right to left. Next, tilt your head sideways, left as far as possible. Return to normal, repeat on right side. Repeat on each side five times. Finally, drop your head forward and swing it around slowly, five times left and five times right.

Before massaging your scalp, try massaging neck and shoulders first to help release general tensions. If you can, get a friend to lend a vigorous hand. With or without friendly assistance, once the tensions from your neck and shoulders have been released, concentrate on the scalp. With thumbs placed above the ears and fingertips outstretched over the scalp, exert gentle pressure, beginning at the base of the scalp. Rotate fingers gradually, moving upward and over the entire scalp. This will help to eliminate tensions that may be slowing down blood circulation to the scalp. In using your fingertips, be careful not to scratch your crown with any sharp fingernails. If hair is extremely damaged, massaging offers a more beneficial means of stimulation than does brushing.

Proper Combing

You've heard the lyrics "Remember that rainy morning, I threw you out, with nothin' but a fine-tooth comb. . ." Well, now you can stop crying the blues. It's an absolute fact that for hair care a wide-toothed comb is far better than a fine-toothed comb. A fine-toothed comb may possibly keep hair clean, but generally pulls out more hair than it cleans.

Those who believe in true naturalism go so far as to say nothing but a tortoise-shell comb will do. (Speert's tortoise-shell comb No. 15 is a really good buy at $2.) Make sure the teeth of your comb are smooth and rounded and avoid metal combs as they create static. Furthermore, metal teeth are apt to be too sharp and harsh to precious hair strands. The moment a tooth breaks off, discard the comb; otherwise you will snag and tear your valuable hair.

To comb, start from the bottom up, in a downward direction. This method will get out the snarls without taking out any hair. Once your hair is tangle-free, comb from the part down.

Combing is a minor stimulant when compared to brushing and massaging, but it helps, too, and keeps hair looking nice and neat. Be sure to keep combs, brushes, and fingers clean at all times.

14.
Coloring Your Hair, Dyeing, Retouching

Beautiful hair also means beautiful hair color, the kind you had when you were a carefree ten year old. Unfortunately, discoloration woes come upon all of us sooner or later. Some are the result of time, others the result of chemicals, fumes, and air pollution. Regardless of the cause, color correction can help to add new highlights to both your hair and your life. Mousy browns, fading blondes, and nondescript colors can come alive cosmetically. The most important thing about hair color is naturalness; a new hair color is right if it looks as though it grew on your head. Just because a color looks beautiful on someone else's head does not mean it will complement you. What counts is how the color blends with your skin tones.

We know now that gray hair is generally hereditary; people don't turn gray overnight, except in exceptional cases of rare disease. Recent research has shown that overexposure to x-rays hastens graying. Caucasians are prone to graying more than any other race. By comparison Orientals are seldom bothered by the phenomenon.

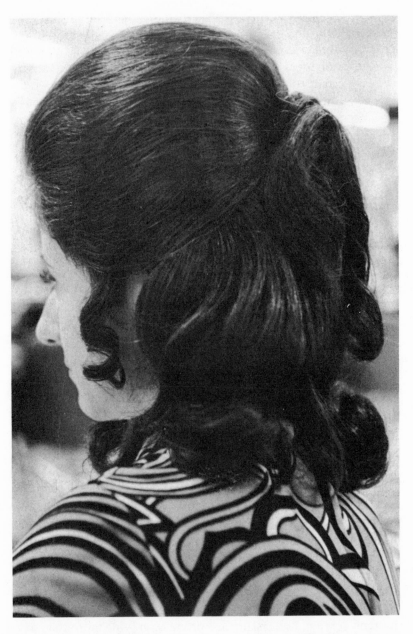

A new hair color is right if it looks as though it grew on your head.

Luckily, when gray hair or other discoloration woes start plaguing your life, you can change things. Hair coloring as an art has improved immeasurably over the last ten years. Still, color can make or break the good looks of your hair. For this reason, it is important to understand the hair-coloring techniques which are available and to know when a professional colorist should do the job. Hair-coloring products must be used carefully, following the manufacturer's instructions step by step.

When hair is to undergo a drastic change, without any question a professional colorist should take over. Often the natural color must be lightened before a new color can be used and this is by no means a do-it-yourself operation. Because natural hair is never one solid color, but rather a blend of several shades, top colorists emphasize blending colors, using three or four shades on the same head, usually light at the front, darker at the back, so that artificially colored hair will reflect light, just as virgin hair does. Harsh darker shades tend to be unflattering to anyone not born a brunette.

Before undertaking a drastic color change, like going from dark brown to Swedish blonde, consider the facts. Do gentlemen really prefer blondes? Do they, in fact, have more fun? Truth is, men date and marry brunettes at the rate of three to one over blondes. By consensus, 99 percent of all the brunettes who have made the switch, revert back to the original, natural color. Brunette doesn't mean just brown; the range of brunette coloring varies from dark blonde to dark black. Brunettes are a majority, redheads a minority. Incidentally, if you are a redhead—beware. Red hair is extremely porous, and dyes can make natural red hair grow back brown.

Before the advent of modern hair-color products, Edgar Cayce, both a prophet and a truth healer, recommended regular doses of the juice of potato peelings as a prescription to maintaining normal hair coloring. To prevent hair from turning gray, or to return it to its natural color, he prescribed that the peelings of Irish potatoes be taken at two meals each day. (Peels could be cooked or uncooked.) Although such prescriptions may have had merit in their day, today modern techniques and products are more readily available than are Irish potatoes.

Visit any cosmetic department or drugstore and you will find three main types of products from which you can choose to alter the color of your hair. The difference between the types lies in their staying power. Temporary rinses last through one shampoo; semipermanent rinses, also known as long-lasting or once-a-month rinses, last through four, six, or eight shampoos; and permanent colors or tints last until new hair growth appears. As is fairly evident, shopping for a hair colorant can be confusing, since there is no agreement on what the different products should be called. Permanent colors are, in fact, dyes, but the word rarely appears on any label, except perhaps on a temporary colorant which proclaims itself as "Not a dye." Dyes are most often called tints, and temporary products are called rinses. To complicate matters more, most companies produce both permanent and temporary products under the same brand name. (Hudnut, Clairol, Roux, Helena Rubenstein, and Marchand, to mention but a few.)

It is also difficult to tell by merely reading a label what type of dye a product may contain. Generally, temporary products contain vegetable coloring in the form of henna, indigo, camomile, sage, nutgall, or saffron. Vegetable coloring is considered a safe means of coloring; however, it is not as effective as coal-tar colors, which is why most manufacturers prefer coal-tar coloring agents even for temporary color rinses. When coal-tar agents are used in permanent or semipermanent tints, Federal regulations require both a cautionary label and directions for making a preliminary skin test against possible allergy. A skin test means applying a bit of the product in the same concentration as will be used when doing the full job on your head. The solution is allowed to dry on a patch of skin—usually behind the ear or on the inside of the elbow—for a period of twenty-four hours. If there is no itching, burning, or other sign of irritation, the product may be used safely.

Permanent colorants sometimes contain a metallic dye. Label warnings are not presently required in connection with metallic dyes. Nevertheless, some labels do state, "For external use only," or "This product contains ingredients which may cause skin irritations on certain individuals, do not apply to broken, open or irritated skin surfaces and discontinue immediately should the skin or scalp become reddened or irritated." The implication is, of course, that metallic dyes if taken internally are poisonous and if applied to damaged skin may lead to systemic poisoning. If directions call for daily applications for a week or longer, so that the color can gradually develop to a particular shade, the product undoubtedly contains a metallic dye. (Your Hair, Bombay Hair Darkener, and RD for Men.)

About 95 percent of all professional hair-dyeing and home-dyeing products contain coal-tar dyes which consist of para-phenylenediamine or related chemicals—also called oxidation dyes, amino dyes, para dyes or peroxide dye. In order to avoid any hazardous chemical reactions which might possibly affect you or your hair, it is important to follow the manufacturer's directions and not to deviate in any way.

Commercial home dyes packaged and designed to appeal to a feminine buyer feature such persuading captions as Magic Moment, Tried and True, Happiness, That's My Color, Nice 'N' Easy, Preference, For Brunettes Only, and Look At Nature, in addition to a host of others. For the gentlemen, Grecian Formula #16, and by Clairol, Great Day—A Man's Way to Remedy Gray, which is perhaps the most persuasive. If you yearn to intensify your own hair color, revive the highlights, or try your hand at being a blonde, here are the types of products available and the type of performance you can expect.

Temporary Rinses

Temporary rinses produce new highlights, but no major color transformation. They help to eliminate minor discoloration and blend gray hair. After one shampoo, the new color effect disappears. Temporary products may come in the form of liquid rinses, powder, crayon, in shampoos, or as applications for use with combs. A temporary-type rinse is a good bet for those who

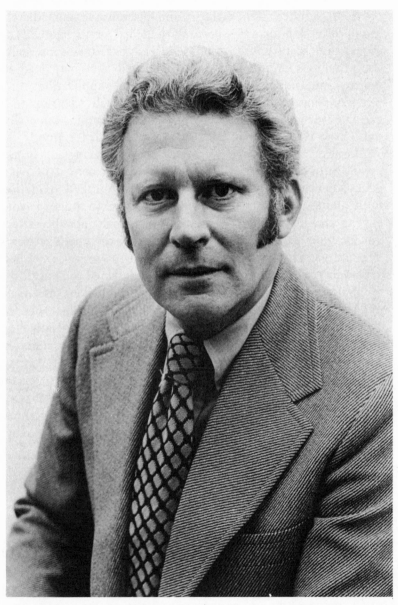

Does he or doesn't he?
Courtesy of Clairol Inc.

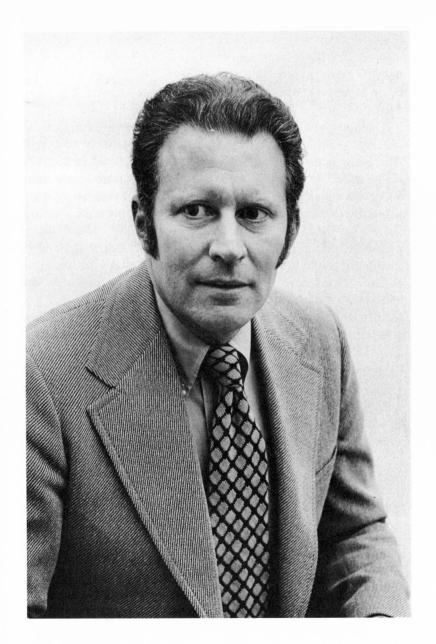

Only his hairdresser knows for sure.

are in an experimental stage. If the results are unflattering, all that is necessary is to shampoo. Since temporary rinses do not produce drastic color changes, it's hard to go wrong. Their main purpose is to add sparkle and highlights with possibly a slight color change—maybe just a little more red, a little more gold, or a little less gray.

Temporary rinses, because of their extra coating, add body to fine hair to make it more manageable and less likely to tangle. When hair is dry, damaged, or split it is wise to avoid use of a color rinse, as the hair is apt to absorb more color than necessary which, in turn, produces an unnatural or harsh color. Under these conditions, the end result is anything but flattering.

How to apply: Simply follow instructions. Some liquid rinses and all powder rinses are diluted in hot water. After shampooing, the liquid solution is poured through the hair until all the strands have been thoroughly covered. Afterwards, the hair is rinsed with cool water until the rinse water appears clear. Insufficient rinsing results in stained pillows, bed sheets, collars, and whatever else your head touches, if an overabundance of dye substance is left on the hair. If you choose a temporary color which comes in a pad form, simply stroke the comb and pad through the hair until the desired effect is obtained—no rinsing is necessary. In all cases, the application of temporary color takes just a few minutes of your time.

Now, if the shade appears fine but is not quite deep enough, next time use more rinse and less water. Leave the rinse on for an extra five minutes before finally rinsing it out. It's best to make a strand test first, so you can get the timing down correctly the first time. Most temporary rinses do not require a skin test. However, if you are hyperallergic, take a skin test and allow twenty-four hours to pass before proceeding.

Temporary-Rinse Color Tips

Graying: Temporary rinses will blend in traces of gray so that gray hairs become less noticeable. A temporary rinse will not transform gray hair into a new color, but can also help to eliminate yellow tones and add a smoky tone to salt-and-pepper gray. Temporary rinses can also add a radiantly silver effect to an overall gray head of hair.

Brunettes: A blonde rinse gives golden highlights; a red shade adds red or auburn highlights; brown tones intensify brown hair and help blend in gray strands and streaks. To liven up medium to dark hair, use a chestnut-tone rinse that will add rich red highlights to your hair.

Blondes: Any color of temporary rinse will affect blonde hair color—light shades will intensify the natural color and even out any slight discolorations; darker shades will add varying intensities of red highlights depending upon the hair's original lightness.

Previously Tinted or Lightened Hair: A temporary ash-blonde rinse will help tone down brassy tones. It will also help to stretch out the time period between touch ups. If bleach has been used previously, dilute the rinse as hair is apt to be overly receptive to color. A strand test is advisable so as to eliminate any unpleasant surprises later on.

Semipermanent Rinses

Semipermanent rinses intensify, highlight, blend gray, and disguise discoloration. They accomplish the same effects as temporary rinses only on a longer, more intensive basis. After four to six shampoos, the new color gradually fades away.

How to apply: Semipermanent rinses are applied in the same manner as temporary rinses; that is, the color solution is applied to freshly shampooed hair. All strands must be completely saturated with the rinse, but it should not be rubbed into the scalp. Semipermanent-color rinses should be rinsed out after a period of approximately twenty minutes. Semipermanent coloring does not interfere with regular barber or salon visits. You can do your own homework and still visit the professionals for styling if that is your style.

Semipermanent Color Tips

If your hair is dry or damaged in any way, avoid using a semipermanent rinse, as hair may overabsorb color. If your hair is in good condition after coloring and you wish to give yourself or get a salon permanent you may do so, providing you allow at least two weeks to pass and remember to precondition your hair with a cream or oil treatment before permanenting. Since permanented hair is more absorbent than normal hair, for even shading, omit coloring porous ends until the very end of your coloring session. Color effects are the same as designated for temporary rinses; they merely last longer.

Permanent Tints

Permanent tints actually change the color of your hair. They can darken or lighten or cover gray on a "permanent" basis, or, in other words, until new hair grows out. Whether packaged as permanent tints, dyes, or creme tints—premixed, push button, mix yourself, or salon prepared—they are essentially all alike. Since the change is permanent, selection of a flattering shade is all important. If in doubt, try a temporary rinse in the same shade first. If you like the effect, plan to use a permanent tint the following week.

When making a color selection, choose a shade slightly lighter if you are in the market for a younger look. Avoid jet blacks unless your hair is naturally jet. A preliminary strand test will allow you to avoid any unpleasant color surprises.

Remember to consider your skin tone. Olive skin looks best when hair is medium to dark brown, with gold highlights added. Ruddy or red skin tones look best with ash-blonde hair coloring. Practically any shade will be flattering to those with fair skin. In all cases, do not tint hair that is dry unless it has first been thoroughly lubricated with an oil treatment and a strand test has been taken to ensure good results.

How to apply: Do not shampoo prior to coloring, unless hair has a heavy buildup of hair spray. Permanent tints are to be applied to dry hair *only*. Follow manufacturer's instructions regarding mixing of dye solution. Color mixture may be dabbed on, sprayed on, or shampooed in, depending on the product which is used. It must, in any case, be applied evenly for perfect results. After a period of twenty to thirty minutes, the tint is removed by means of rinsing or shampooing according to the maker's instructions. Before permanent tinting at home, take a skin test for possible allergic reaction to the dyeing chemicals. If after 24 hours results are satisfactory, you may proceed safely. Follow the instructions of the manufacturer.

Most home products have now been streamlined to the point where all you need do is assemble the proper equipment—a towel, a clock or timer, plastic gloves, and the color products, which usually consist of peroxide developer and a color agent which are to be combined according to the directions. The entire mixture is then applied—usually from a plastic squeeze-bottle applicator—and worked throughout the hair in the same manner as if you were shampooing. The color mixture should be allowed to develop for approximately 20 minutes. The next stage generally requires adding a little water until a rich lather develops, which then must be rinsed out thoroughly until the rinse water runs clear. One hour is all you need allow for your color session.

Permanent Tint Color Tips

Too Light: If the new permanent color comes out lighter than what you want, a weak solution of a temporary rinse will help intensify the color. Be sure to make a strand test to determine result.

Too Dark: If your new permanent color is darker than you desire, a solution of one-part peroxide and one-part conditioning oil used several times will help lift out excess color, and will soften the hair at the same time.

For Brunettes: Brunettes sometimes find that after using a blond tint their hair has more red highlights than desired. In order to eliminate this brassiness, bleaching or toning may be required. Either process is best left in the hands of professionals.

For Blondes: A blond tint helps add pretty highlights to deep-blond or drab-blond colors. A special shampoo mixture of one-part twenty-volume peroxide, one-part special drabbing tint color, and one-part shampoo will help to subdue brassiness. Another way to combat brassiness is to use a temporary rinse.

Brassiness: The cause of brassiness if often due to the overcoloring which results when hair is too porous. When hair is dry and overporous, have it trimmed. If your hair has oxidized to an unpleasant color, next time select a toner close to the shade you began with, mix and apply per instructions given by the manufacturer.

Handling the Touch Up

If you have made a radical color change, in order to maintain even color, retouch only the new growth. Section hair and apply the tint to partings with a plastic applicator or cotton-swab applicator. Work the solution into newly grown hairs. Do not overlap on previously dyed hair. Avoid combing the new dye through the hair. Get a friend to help you retouch the back part of your hair until you yourself become an expert or unless you visit an expert. On the average, when there is a drastic color change, roots must be touched up every four weeks and a complete redyeing is necessary two or three times a year.

On those occasions when you may be too rushed for a legitimate touch up, try using a color pencil to blend in gray hairs so that they will match your tint color—providing it is in the red-brown family. Unfortunately, light color-crayon pencils do not have any effect on darker hair colors.

Bleaching

Bleaching is another method of changing hair color. This is usually accomplished with hydrogen peroxide. The initial bleaching requires a good number of sessions lasting several hours each, with frequent and prolonged applications of peroxide. Color transformation ranges from jet black to brown to red to gold to yellow to pale yellow. To successfully achieve a delicate blond or red shade after bleaching, a second process is required. Color toner, a form of dye which penetrates the lightened hair shaft, must be applied to instill new subtle coloring. The degree of lightening required for the desired shade is described on the toner package. Bleached hair often suffers loss of luster, becomes dry, and is extremely susceptible to damage when subsequent dyeing or permanenting takes place.

Bleaching should never be a home operation and, in general, should be avoided altogether, as the treatment is excessively harsh to hair and once begun must be kept up monthly. If you are a blonde naturally and wish to lighten your hair just a bit, the likelihood of damage is slight, since excessive bleaching will not be required to lighten the hair. In other words, so long as you do not overbleach, the chances of damage are minimal. Brunettes, on the other hand, can avoid disastrous hair problems by avoiding bleaching or use of tint color which require prebleach treatments.

Frosting, tipping and streaking are lightening variations which give a brightening effect to the entire head by lightening selected hair strands. To accomplish this, a two-part bleach-toner process is used. Frosting gives an overall sunlit look by lightening individual strands throughout all the hair. Tipping gives a sunlit effect by lightening selected hairs surrounding the face. Streaking is the lightening and toning of six to ten adjacent hair strands on either one or both sides of the face. Lightening variations are most successful when left to the expert hands of the professionals. Home preparations are chancy in untrained hands and are for use only on virgin hair.

Never use bleach or permanent chemicals on top of frosted, tipped or streaked hair.

Important Color Pointers

1. Following a good hair-care program is vital during the summertime and especially so for heads on a tinting or dyeing schedule. If hair is dried out and overlightened by the sun, it becomes porous and color winds up uneven. To avoid this give your hair extra protection and the care it needs during the hot summer months. Before getting entrenched, remember, not every woman looks good in light-colored hair.

2. If you are determined to lighten your hair, consider variations ranging from pale to dark blond, through ash, honey, and red shades. Select a shade that will flatter your complexion. As the years fly by, skin tones change and a very bright-colored shade may appear harsh and unbecoming. Under these conditions, a natural blonde is advised to maintain her original color, not go lighter. A brunette turning blonde needs restraint, going just a few shades lighter. For many brunettes, the best answer is to highlight the hair by adding brighteners, by merely frosting, tipping, or streaking a few select strands.

3. Both bleached and tinted hair require special treatment. For example, neglecting to use hair-care products specially designed for use for bleached or color-treated hair can lead to unattractive, unnatural color or to a drab overall unflattering color. If you color your hair, choose a shampoo made specially for color-treated hair, so as to leave the hair-color tones you like intact. Always follow with a creme rinse that will help keep your hair in good condition. If your hair snarls or mats when it is wet, as lightened hair sometimes does, use a conditioning creme rinse. Every two weeks use a one-minute conditioner with protein to strengthen and condition your hair strands from end to end. For lightened or bleached hair, apply a twenty-minute conditioner at least once a month, and if you set your

hair, use a conditioner with hair-setting action in one of the three strengths your hair type requires. There are especially gentle setting lotions for color-lightened hair. At all times, you should hide tinted, bleached, frosted, or tipped hair from the sun and wind.

4.   Never use any hair-coloring product on your brows or lashes unless that is what the product is specifically designed for. Using hair dye on brows or lashes can easily burn or damage delicate eye tissues.

5.   Before tinting your hair, take the precautionary measure of coating forehead, neck, and cheeks with vasoline or a cleansing cream. This will eliminate the need for rough scrubbing if any permanent dye gets on your skin; if it does, tissue off immediately.

By knowing what color methods are available, and how they can be made to work for you, the opportunity of adding new sparkle to both your locks and your life lies within your reach.

15.
The Male Hair Revolution – Today's Trend

The man of today purchases his own hair sprays, buys his own shampoo, and his own hair-color products—in addition to a complete line of male grooming aids.

Today's man realizes that his hair is his own personal calling card; it can suggest his social station, his political allegiance, even his membership in a particular group, and, in some societies, his sexual preferences. The male of today thoroughly comprehends why women have for so long willingly spent time and quantities of money on making their hair beautiful. He is willing to devote as much or more to keeping his hair.

In our present society, finding an old-fashioned barber shop is next to impossible. More often barbers are referred to as hair stylists, hair designers, hair clinicians, or masculine coiffeurists. Slowly but surely, ye old barber shops are being replaced by men's hair studios where sophisticated stylists specialize in long hair, creative cutting, scientific shampooing, hair coloring, straightening, scalp treatments, and hair pieces. According to data from Hollywood Joe's Hairpiece Co., Inc., men get just as

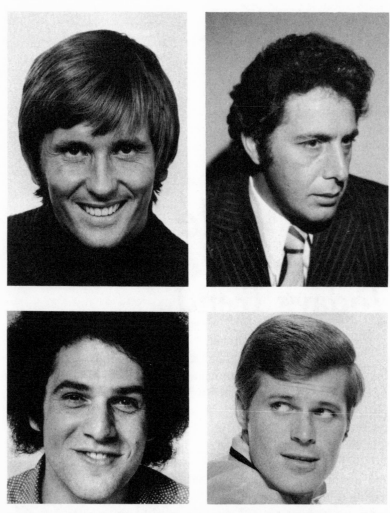

Today's man realizes that hair is his own personal calling card.
Courtesy of Clairol Inc.

much of a psychological uplift from a hairpiece as do women. Hollywood Joe's advertisements proclaim that a balding, gray-haired nondescript fellow can be turned into a superstar through hirsute magic. Regardless of which head treatment is involved, men are absolutely wild over their new freedom, and indulge in the world of hair care with possibly even more enthusiasm than do their female counterparts.

A recent copy of *Professional Barber Magazine* reports that over 160 firms now manufacture a full line of men's grooming aids. As far as hair products are concerned, men give their own stamp of approval to hair dyes, dryers, teasing combs, hair nets, and sprays—and are willing to pay scalpers' prices. Two dollars for a haircut is a rare happening; most men prefer a styling job, and are willing to go as high as twenty dollars for a trim—which clearly points out the difference between ye old barbering and today's hair styling. But instead of dying by the wayside, as one might suppose, more and more shops are making the transition from barber to stylist. Posters sprouting up in barber shops across the country, exemplify the transition from old to new:

WHEN WE SAY WE'RE HAIR STYLISTS, WE'RE NOT JUST GIVING YOU A FANCY NAME FOR "BARBER."

There's a difference between getting your hair cut and getting your hair styled. Come in and we'll define that difference as it relates to your own hair. There's no obligation.

When you say, "Take just a little bit off," we take just a little bit off. We know that unless we make you happy the first time, there'll be no second time.

HOW TO CHOOSE A GOOD BARBER WITHOUT RISKING A BAD HAIRCUT: WATCH THE GUY WORK ON SOMEONE ELSE BEFORE HE WORKS ON YOU. COME IN. SIT DOWN AND WATCH A GOOD BARBER WORK.

DON'T LET YOUR HAIR GROW ALL BY ITSELF!
Some men look terrific when they let their hair grow.
Because they don't try to grow it singlehandedly. They
come in regularly and have it styled. And shaped and
layered. And blended. And trained.

Then there are the other guys who, when they let their
hair grow, just look like they need a haircut because they
try to grow it alone. And it grows out of control.

The moral is, if you want your long hair to look great,
don't make the mistake of staying away from us too long.

WHY LONG HAIR SHOULD BE CUT AS OFTEN AS
SHORT HAIR: Most guys think long hair needs less
tending to than short hair.

Fact is, long hair requires more because it has a
tendency to look wild unless it's shaped and styled
regularly.

And because long hair gets to be too long unless it's
trimmed regularly.

It isn't the length of your hair that should determine
how often you visit us.

It's how good you want it to look.

The attitude represented by these posters is indicative of the
tive of the headway that is taking place on a nationwide basis.

To understand what has happened, you need only overhear
what goes on inside the average barber shop as a patron gives his
barber instructions. When a man says cut an eighth of an inch
off, he's not fooling. One iota more, and he won't be back
again. It's come to the point where men consult with their
barber, or stylist as he is more aptly called, as if he were a
stockbroker. And there's good reason. The range of styles for
men has become almost as endless as those for women. A man
can go to any length—short, medium, or long—all depending on
how he prefers to express himself. The end result—men wind up
spending as much time and experimenting being curried as do
women, with almost as many choices at their disposal.

A visit to the salon of Monsieur Jacques, 14 East 56th Street in New York City, offers the plush option of giving a man his pick of comfy chairs or his own private booth, equipped with telephone. The real enticement for many prominent heads is Jacques' delectable remedial shampoos concocted of vegetables and fruits. Before preparing the remedial wash, he determines which vegetable or fruit to use by analyzing the customer's hair condition. Avocado for very dry hair, carrot for medium dry, banana for dry, celery for oily. Cabbage and egg, too, are sometimes combined for extra lush benefits. Jacques crushes the vegetables in a machine and mixes the juices with a neutral soap; no alcohol is ever used. His interest is in maintaining a healthy head of hair, not in recovering the heads of bald men.

Elliot Nonas, president of Penthouse For Men, is proud of his establishment and its "Second Head of Hair." If a man has inherited the dominant genes for baldness, Nonas says, he's going to be bald—and under the present conditions, no miracle is going to change the inevitable. Massages, special oils, brushing, etc., can only help the hair that exists; but it won't bring back lost hair resulting from the male-pattern baldness. The Second Head of Hair is Nonas' trade name for what he believes to be the most undetectable, easiest-to-live-with hair replacement on the market. It's so remarkably real that the nomenclature *second head of hair* is a natural. The parade of Penthouse customers, together with true affidavits, attest to the advancement and naturalness of today's hairpieces.

Stefan Forino, award-winning hairstylist of Le Tapis men's salon fame, is the creator of a remarkable hairpiece which he calls "Signature." Fornio, bald since age twenty-two, has traveled extensively, studying the adaptability of different types of hair, and has researched the differing manufacturing processes. His resultant Signature is "as much a reflection of a man's personality as the way he signs his name." Each Forino hairpiece is specially made for the wearer. At Forino's salon, hairpieces range in size from a diameter of one inch to a length of seven inches. They are priced accordingly; a simple hairpiece begins at $25. The French name, *Le Tapis*, Forino explains, "means 'the rug,' and was selected as our name because if a man needs a rug, he won't be charged for wall-to-wall carpeting."

At Rudel's Salon in New York, the emphasis for men is on highly individualistic styling. Each customer is treated as a distinctly unique individual, and no two men ever walk out sporting the exact same haircut or the same styling. Whether in the Afro department or in the straight department, the look always belongs individually and distinctively to the wearer.

Georgette Briand (22 East 72nd Street in New York City, and 9601 Wilshire Boulevard in Los Angeles) is one of the few women who gives equal attention to men's hair-care problems. Men, she states, start losing their hair around the age of eighteen, but don't begin to notice the loss until several years later. Caring at an early age, she asserts, helps to avoid or lessen hair problems at a later age. Madame Briand compares dyeing hair to the dying leaves of a plant—once the leaf turns yellow, it's dead even though it may remain on the branch. Like a plant, dead hairs may hang on—but they cannot be saved. Her interest lies in making way for the growth of new hairs. Madame Briand's treatment for falling hair is not geared for problems stemming from such inside jobs as nervous conditions or ill health. Her answer to male hair loss is "Etheirologie," a hair-and-scalp nourishing treatment utilizing natural products— herbs, flowers, fruits, plants, and eggs—to fertilize and stimulate hair follicles.

Although she does not believe she can grow hair on a bald head, she can maintain existing hair by keeping the blood circulating properly, so that the scalp receives proper nourishment. Her treatment is geared to nourishing hair-growing roots.

Madame Briand's campaign is an eight-point program: (1) stimulation of circulation around the hair follicles to facilitate hair growth—to accomplish this she applies lemon, flower pollen, and fruit extract in a vitamin liquid; (2) massage of neck and shoulders to help promote the passage of blood to the scalp; (3) disinfecting and stimulating pores by directing ozone-vapor steam onto the head and then applying a cream composed of egg yolk, mineral oil, apple and grape pits, crushed bone marrow, and Panama wood; (4) for sheen and luster, hair is thereafter rinsed, and a plant pack applied consisting of dried herbs, honey, and water; (5) an herbal shampoo of pure, natural products is used to cleanse the hair; (6) a nourishing lemon-base tonic is applied to stimulate new hair growth; (7) an ultraviolet comb is run through the hair to further deep massage and stimulate circulation; and (8) the end result—healthy, great-looking hair.

Madame Briand's whole treatment costs $13.50; $15 for women.

Armand, Los Angeles beauty-school owner and former barber-beautician claims his new Hair Trigger program helps men grow hair. With the assistance of an Indian mystic, astrology charts, natural vitamins, and the formula of a deceased Bulgarian king, Armand has developed a line of hair-raising products including scalp-treatment creams, food supplements, vitamins, and shampoos.

The original formula, bequeathed to an acquaintance by a dying gypsy king, called for such quaint ingredients as bear fat, extract of horse's mane, and whale sperm. One might well believe that the gypsy king had memorized the secrets of the papyrus papers which, thousands of years B.C., called for almost the same hair-raising ingredients. Armand, upon learning of the formula, became intrigued; and, after a battery of home tests, augmented the ingredients, adding vitamins A, B complex, and E. Ultimately, he arrived at his own preparation, which he calls Hair Trigger Formula 6.

Armand offers this explanation for the success which he claims: "The Hair Trigger program nurtures hair follicles beneath the scalp, and eventually helps them to grow. Many people think the loss of hair means the actual hair follicle is dead. We've discovered it is merely like a seed living dormant under the skin. It can be brought back to life if proper care is taken."

It would seem that out of a little seed, Armand has raised some mighty big acorns. Such notables as John Wayne are now

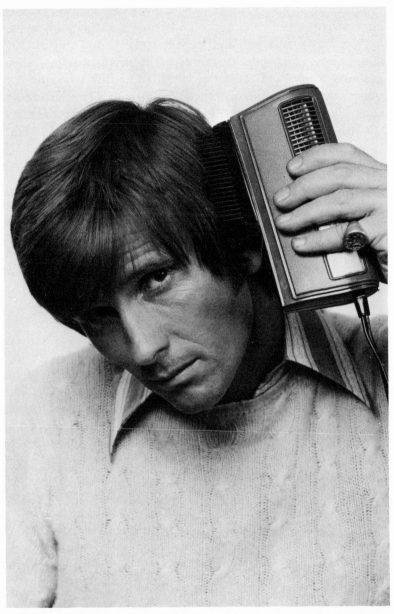

From every appearance, the man's beauty scene is here to stay. Courtesy of Clairol Inc.

said to endorse Armand's products together with his Hair Trigger program.

The opportunities for men are, without question, reaching mind-boggling proportions. From every appearance, the man's beauty scene is here to stay.

16.
The
Beauty-Parlor
Scene

Just a few short years ago, a healthy proportion of beauty-conscious women began boycotting beauty parlors. The reason for the move was simply that, instead of receiving tender, loving, hair care for which they were paying top dollar, beauty-parlor visits were frustrating confrontations. Often careless operators yanked and pulled curlers out so rapidly that one woman swore half her hair was still left on the rollers. Hair was rolled so tightly by some, customers complained of aching scalps; other women complained they were being treated like cattle, herded from a shampoo trough, branded by rollers and, to add insult to injury, left to pasture under a hair dryer turned up full blast. Women began to tire of seeing their hair go down the drain and a silent majority simply quit the beauty-shop routine in favor of treating and caring for their own hair. And lots of people grew lots of hair all by themselves.

When a decline in business became obvious, the industry was forced to reappraise its techniques and overall attitudes. In the end, improvements were seen in both areas generally charac-

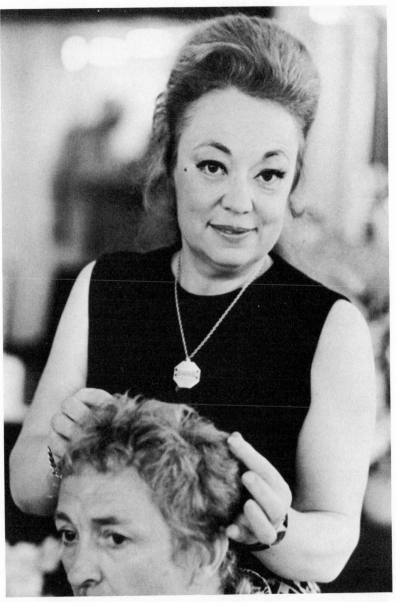

At her hair and scalp clinic, Georgette Briand specializes in "Etheirologie."

terized by greater care and a greater respect for the patron. Today, the number of reliable professionals specializing in the handling of long hair and in promoting its growth stretches from coast to coast. Some of the best experts are located in smog-polluted areas, where the need for air and hair-care help is greatest.

On top of the list is Georgette Briand's Hair-and-Scalp Clinics, mentioned in the preceding chapter, designed to help men and women recover the natural beauty of hair is a return to nature through organics, singeing, and Etheirologie.

Other top names include Don Lee, famous New York problem solver, located at 50 West 57th Street in New York City; Stephen Ball, Organic Hair Care Center, Mill Valley, California; George Michael of Madison Avenue, whose cry is: "If you have long hair, we love you; if you want to grow it long, we help you!"; Guy Paris of Paris West Hairstylists, 157 West 72nd Street in New York City—here the scientific approach is stressed, together with product knowledge and individual customer education, and an emphasis on organics, microanalysis, and home hair-care techniques that entice both the long-haired and the short-haired; Rudel, well-known stylist of Rudel's Salon For Men and Women, 71 Lexington Avenue in New York City, whose motto is: "Look to the top!" and whose following includes such celebrities as Carmen MacRae, Leslie Uggams, Nancy Wilson, and 90 percent of all black models in New York; Gene Shacove in Los Angeles; Valerie Chiz in Hollywood; Rich Ross of Indianapolis; Larry Caffey of San Francisco; and Louis Gignac of Louis-Guy D'Coiffeurs in New York City.

Finding An Expert

If you want to learn how to handle your own hair, or even if you want to turn the task over to the professionals, you must first find an expert. Today, there is a whole new generation of hairdressers from which to choose. Remember, though, that even in the hands of an expert, success comes through experience; so give the expert sufficient time to become familiar with your hair. Your hair may have its own little idiosyncrasies which, by now, you accept as normal. Watch what the experts do and then practice at home in front of your own mirror.

Finding the right person may take a little time. A good shortcut is to get a personal recommendation from a friend. When checking out the tip, be sure to mention your friend's name, if that's how you found your way to the salon. Bear in mind that miracles don't necessarily happen in one session. A new hairdresser, even the best expert, has to get to know your hair.

If you're new in town and don't know which way to turn, pay a visit to the most reputable department store—it undoubtedly has an equally good beauty salon inside. Whenever making an appointment with a new salon, beware of dead giveaways. For example, never trust a salon that offers to squeeze you in—quality work can't be rushed. If a salon tells you, "All our operators are experts," keep looking, even if it means traveling out of your way to find another salon!

When you go away on vacation, finding the best hairdresser can also pose problems unless you take the time to plan ahead. More than likely your home hairdresser will be able to recommend a reliable salon or even a hairdresser. Names can be obtained by checking a professional hairdressing association. Perhaps friends who may live in the vacation area can steer you in the right direction. In any case, if you are partial to a particular product, let the hairdresser know early, preferably when you call for your first appointment. Trip time is no time to begin experimenting. Try to avoid major operations such as hair coloring, permanenting, or cutting.

Hair expert Mr. Kenneth offers sensible hair travel tips for women on the go. Obviously, the simpler your hair style, the simpler its care will be. Hairpieces are a tremendous boon when traveling; the latest creations can be rolled up, packed, then brushed into style again in moments. The most useful hairpieces to take along are wigs and a fall or two. Since a fall is generally straight, it requires next to no upkeep. A simple, long, thick braid to wear after swimming can be extremely attractive and very handy.

If you are adventurous, you may want to have your hair done in a new style by a new hairdresser in a brand-new town or city. Look around at the styles other women are wearing. As long as they are atractive and do not call for a drastic cut, the change can be enjoyable. In some instances, a crowded itinerary may not allow time for hairdresser visits. If this is the case, be sure to pack a dry shampoo for freshening up your hair, especially if it has a tendency to be oily. Or, pour a little cologne or toilet water on a piece of cotton and wipe it along your hairline. Try parting your hair in small sections and rubbing the damp cotton over your exposed scalp, not over the entire hair strand. This will also help to remove some of the oil and dirt and make your hair feel clean.

If you are dependent on certain products or practices, don't hesitate to take your own shampoo, rinses, combs, and brushes, etc. You may even want to take along your own water. In England, for example, the water is perfect; in France it is terrible. Soap has a tendency to cling to the hair and a bottle of natural spring water used for the final rinse can make all the difference in the world.

Wherever and whenever, keep your eye on the stylist, so you can try to duplicate the job yourself whenever you want to try your hand. If you like the finished product, snap a polaroid picture and bring it with you when you return for your next visit, so the stylist can give a repeat performance.

Knowing the right terminology gives you a good head start at any salon. A haircut or a restyle generally means a different look from what you have. A trim is less expensive. It doesn't change your basic style; it is just a neatening process. A set refers to rolling rollers in your hair and putting pin curls where they belong. A shampoo, often priced in combination with a set, can range from a regular plain shampoo to an ultradeluxe herbal or organic treatment. Generally, if you bypass the shampoo, the cost of the set goes up. A rinse is an extra treatment that conditions, manages, or adds highlights to your hair. A comb-out is a redo of your hair—brushing, combing, and final arrangement, without a shampoo or a set. On special occasions, you may want your hairdresser to refinish your style, if an occasion crops up in between your normal salon visits.

Styling

Hairdos once worn exclusively by the young are now fashionable for the chic set. Young people, it seems, set the pace and everyone else follows the best they can, including those of more mature years. For both sexes, curly hair is better than straight and long hair is better than short. The very ultimate in styling—matching his-and-her haircuts; the question sometimes being, "Is she, or isn't she?" In the most fashionable nightclubs and discotheques, pageboy bobs are the rage—regardless of sex. In view of the present scene, what is said hereafter applies to both men and women.

Start with the right haircut. Artful cutting is best left in the hands of an expert. Remember, a good haircut will survive even the worst set. A reputable salon has earned its good reputation, however, even in the best salon, some stylists are better than others. When making an appointment, request a stylist who specializes in haircuts. A cut and styling by a top professional can cost $30, or more, but good results are well worth the expenditure. If possible bring a picture of the style you prefer. Don't visit a new hairdresser without some idea of what you want. Talk about your hair and how it behaves. Discuss the pros and cons of the cut and style you are considering. If the hairdresser doesn't feel your choice is right for you, take his advice.

Blunt Cutting

Blunt cutting means cutting straight across the base of the hair with either a scissors or a razor. Hair is cut to one length all

Three Variations of a Blunt Cut (Figures 1, 2, and 3)

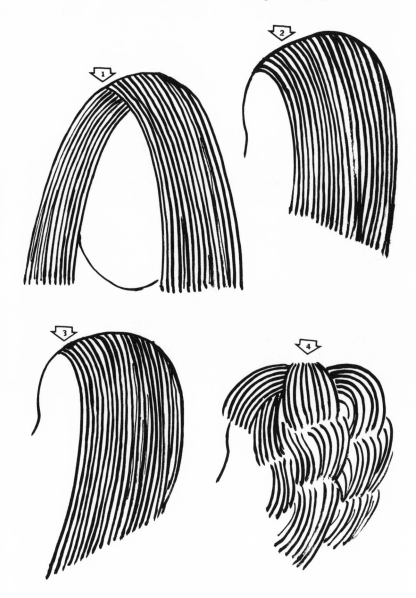

around, whether it be chin length, shoulder length, or longer. Blunt cuts are especially effective for hair that needs extra bulk, such as fine, thin, soft, or split-end hair. A blunt cut helps to play down extra-curly hair. Simple styles, too, may call for blunt cutting. Because of the extra weight this type of cuts adds to the base of hair; swing-length styles may also require a blunt cut. A scissor cut is always preferable to a razor cut. Hair that is blunt cut by a razor tends to be sliced at an angle, thereby exposing more of the inner hair shaft and allowing moisture to escape from the hair. Coloring or permanenting hair which is razor-sliced often leads to greater potential harm, as more of the inner hair shaft is exposed. Variations on the blunt cut—hair may be blunt cut with the back portion of hair blunt cut shorter than sides, or hair can blunt cut with sides shorter than the back.

Tapering

Tapering means cutting across hair ends at an angle. This, too, can be done with a scissors or a razor. Natural curly or wavy hair reacts best to tapering. Since the angle of this cut exposes more of the inner portion of the hair shaft, tapering leaves hair more open to possible injury. Using a scissor rather than a razor cut, lessens this hazard.

Layering

Layering means cutting hair in layers at a succession of varying lengths. It is today's vogue look. Most professionals prefer to blunt cut the layers at an established and uniform length; if one layer is three inches long, then all the layers will be approximately three inches long. The word layering is currently described in various terms: Shag, the Gypsy, even, unflatteringly, the Ape. They are all simply layered cuts. The overall look can be long, short, or medium depending upon the length of the layers. Often layering is combined with tapering to achieve short, ruffled, wavy or curly styles. Curly hair most easily adapts to layering. The look is great; however, getting back to a single-length style is not easy. Growing hair to one length requires patience, fortitude and frequent trims.

Most expert stylists cut hair according to the direction in which it grows and, for better control, usually prefer to cut while hair is wet. Rudel has a super technique. Dry ends are snipped off while the hair is still dry; then the hair is wet and cut once more, this time, the curl factor is taken into account. While hair is still damp, he cuts a third time for shape. Whether you're dry, wet, or only slightly soggy, your hair looks tops.

If you have ever wondered whether shaving your hair will make it grow in thicker, the answer is it won't. New hair only feels thicker because the blunt new ends have a coarse quality when they start peeking through the skin. Hairs that have not been shaved have a more gently tapered end and so feel softer to the touch. Actually, the diameter of each hair remains the same whether it has been shaved or not.

The best length for your hair is partially determined by the texture of your hair. Fine, flyaway hair has a tendency to look thin. To create a look of bulk, fine hair ideally should be worn no longer than chin length and should be blunt cut. Medium-textured hair that holds a set and behaves itself can be worn at almost any length, depending upon the styling. Coarse hair is often unruly and may be hard to curl. A long blunt cut will help keep it manageable and hold the ends properly in place. Curly hair, regardless of texture or quantity, should not be cut too short, as any sudden humidity will encourage it to frizz and look unkempt and out of control. Wild, too-thick hair can look prettier and more manageable with layering, which helps to put all the weight in the right place.

How often you need to have your hair cut will depend in large measure on the length you prefer and on the hair style selected. Short hair worn close to the head may have to be trimmed every three or four weeks. Medium-length hair can go up to six weeks before cutting. Long hair may only need a trim every three to four months. Remember, if you are going from long hair to short hair, the change can take just a few short minutes; reversing the process, however, can take months, if not years, to recoup. You must allow approximately a month for half an inch of new hair growth. Simple mathematics predicts just how long it will be before your cropped hair can be expected to hit shoulder length.

Although a poor cut can be frustrating, don't stand there tearing your hair out. Manage your hair while it grows out. Hide unevenly cut sections by curling longer strands over uneven parts. If hair is too short all over, try shaping it around large rollers, and camouflage the whole mistake with tousled curls. If one side is shorter than the other, curl the long side to match, or try teasing the longer strands to look shorter. Sometimes an asymmetrical look can be achieved by sweeping the short hair back and fluffing the longer locks wide at the other side. Uneven bangs can become an asset by merely brushing them casually to one side.

If you want your layered hair to grow out into one length but don't want to spend six months looking like a sheepdog, take the advice of Philip Mason of the Vidal Sassoon Salon in New York—for the first two months let it grow until you can't stand it anymore; then, and only then, have the bottom layer of hair trimmed to even the line. Don't have crown hair cut at all for about six months, but do keep trimming the back bottom layer of hair every two months, so that an overall even effect takes place. At this point hair can go for roughly another four months before a final trim is required. By now your original short shag will be close to chin length. To get through those frustrating periods of waiting for crown hair to grow long, try controlling the situation by pulling a thick clump of hair together at the top of the head and clipping it back with a barrette, or tie a pretty ribbon around the section of hair.

Styling Approaches

There are several approaches to finding your best hair style. The simplest and quickest is to have an expert show you the hairdo possibilities for both your hair type and facial features. Barring professional assistance, begin by experimenting in front of your mirror. One classic trick which helps is accomplished by working up a good shampoo lather on the hair and scalp and then experimenting. Don't be afraid to push your hair around; high, low, full, angle it, curve it, slant it. Of the almost unlimited ways there are to wear your hair, one shape, one line, and one look is tailor-made for you, and promises to show off your best features. A good hair style accentuates the positives and eliminates the negatives. A center part and width at the crown make close-set eyes appear more widely spaced. Eyes, too, can be made to look larger, even the nose you sometimes hate can suddenly seem pert, with the right style. A large face can be made to appear more delicate. A prominent forehead can be disguised; so can a receding chin. Keep experimenting. When you find a look you like, analyze it, memorize the lines, and aim for the same look after the shampoo suds are gone.

Here's a trick for the nonbashful. Visit a local department store with a good wig department. Try on various styled wigs until you find one that appeals to you. To keep everything in proper perspective, remember that small faces and features should use a hairdo of small proportions. Large faces and features look best in full, fluffy styles. Large or tall individuals seem to have heads too small for their bodies when wearing up-tight, clinging hair styles. The reverse is equally true. A huge hairdo on a small person makes for an awkward top-heavy look. When you find a wig style that truly becomes you, memorize the line and look, and try for the same styling at home.

Often facial structure is the key to finding your best style. Faces fall naturally into six distinctive shapes and certain hair styles are naturally more or less flattering to each shape. Try categorizing the shape of your face and then incorporating the following styling tips:

Oval-shaped: If this is your type, you're in good shape. You can choose and wear practically any hair style, bearing in mind the look you personally prefer. Long and loose or short and fluffy, both can be equally flattering.

Heart-shaped or triangular: A flattering balance can be achieved for heart-shaped faces by keeping hair fairly long, just below the chin line and casually tucking hair behind the ears. A side sweep of bangs can also add a flattering touch. If your hair responds best to short styling and you want to minimize a broad forehead, try a short, curly style with short, straight bangs, together with lightly overlapping curly bangs. Use crisp side waves over the temple areas and a fluffy brush-up tapered look at the nape of the neck.

Oblong: An oblong face finds its own drama when hair is parted on the side and worn in a fluffy, curly style, midlength between chin bone and chin. Avoid lifting hair on top.

Diamond-shaped: If your face is narrow at the temples and jawline, but broad across the cheekbones, try a center part with chin-length hair which can be fluffed out at the ends to give extra width and a flattering balance. For shorter hair styling, try a layered cut with short top and side hair and slightly longer nape hair at the neckline. Add casually fluffy bangs and loose wavy locks over the cheekbone area.

Square: Square faces benefit when the hair is worn at medium length and with ends fluffed up just above the jawline to minimize and soften angles.

Round: A round face gets an extra lift from hair that is added on top to build height. Side hair is best worn short, clinging and curving below the cheeks to make the face seem longer and narrower than its true shape.

Quantity and quality of hair are also keys to finding a falttering style. Hair texture and volume predetermine how your hair will react. Smooth, straight lines work successfully on average and coarse hair. For fine or thin hair, these same styles are likely to be disappointing. Fine, thin, or sparse hair respond better to short, partless, fluffy styles that help make hair look fuller. Coarse hair, cut and shaped by expert hands, can be worn in practically any style. Fine and medium-fine hair very frequently refuses to cooperate with full-length, curly styles. Wavy hair, no matter how slight the wave, always rejects ultrastraight

Facial Shape Determines Which Hair Style Is Best

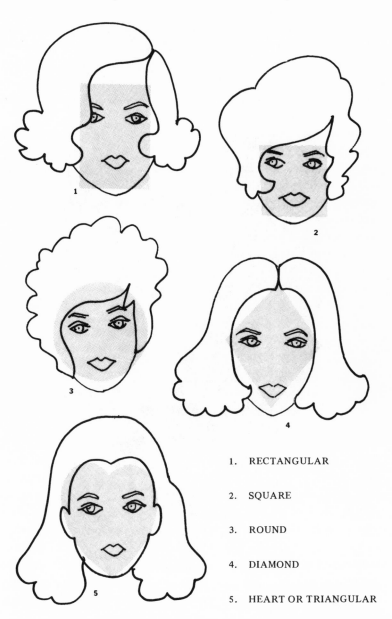

1. RECTANGULAR

2. SQUARE

3. ROUND

4. DIAMOND

5. HEART OR TRIANGULAR

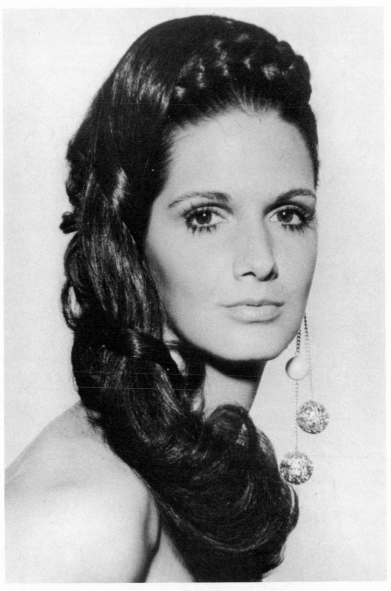

Long hair offers more versatility than does short hair. Courtesy of Clairol Inc.

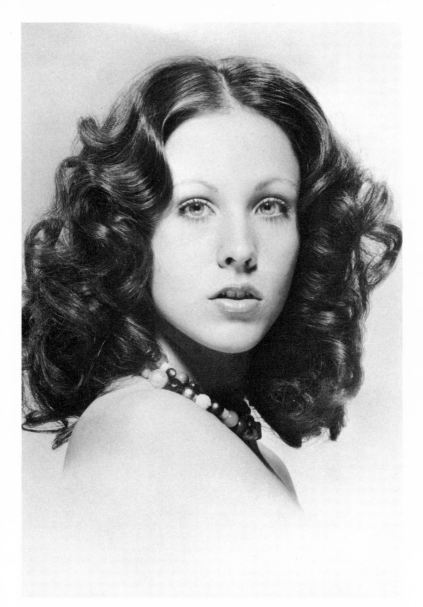

Men have always found loose natural-looking styles sexier than artificial concoctions. Courtesy of Clairol Inc.

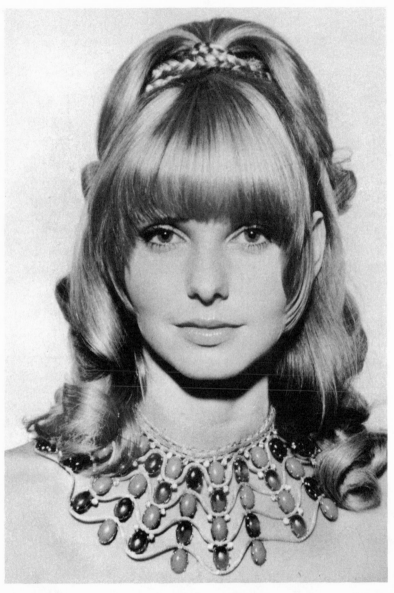

The look today—an expensively achieved casualness of hair styling. Courtesy of Clairol Inc.

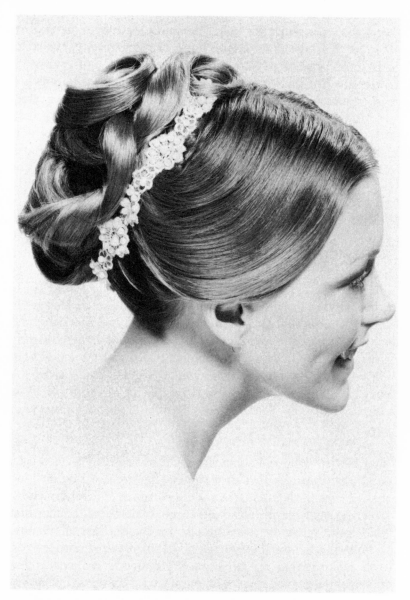

Leather, beads, bows or ribbons are all an indication of you and your personality. Courtesy of Clairol Inc.

styling. To circumvent a cowlick, the best solution is to have hair cut and parted to accommodate the way the hair naturally swirls. If a particular style does not cooperate with the texture of your hair, keep experimenting until you find a style that suits both your facial structure and the texture and volume of your hair. The choice of styles is endless. There is absolutely no point in trying to make your hair do what it cannot characteristically carry out. Although you may be tempted to try to alter the texture of your hair, this should be as a last resort. If you use your head wisely, chances are you need not even consider changing your hair's texture.

Life style should definitely influence hair style. Are you easily bored? Long hair offers more versatility than does short hair. It can be worn up, down, or changed in endless ways by merely changing the part. Not supercrafty with your hair? If you're all thumbs or constantly on the go, choose a style that requires a minimum of fussing. Do you wear glasses? Eyeglasses coupled with the right hair style can be extremely attractive. If you wear your glasses most of the time, keep your hairdo simple and off the face. If you want bangs with your glasses, keep the bangs short and preferably sideswept. Avoid large, dangling earrings and, instead, indulge in eye makeup. How much time can you comfortably allow for your routine of daily styling? If yours is a busy rush-a-day world, simplicity of style will allow you more time to do the things you enjoy rather than fuss with pins, curlers and combs.

Try taking a lesson from today's beautiful people who wear their hair straight and shoulder length or short and shaped via a good professional cut. Get a straight blunt cut if you have no curl, or a layered cut that can be washed and blown dry—both are great bets for people on the go. Remember, though, that what looks great on someone else may spell disaster for you. Despite all the hints, experiment in front of your own mirror, push your hair in all directions until you find the line that enhances your face most. Sometimes by examining a snapshot of yourself you can readily spot where improvements can be made or what you're now doing wrong. Looking at photographs of other individuals who share a similar facial structure may also give you a new lead. No matter how great it may look, if you want to avoid a receding hairline, possible hair loss, or even balding, do not pull hair tightly back into either a bun or a ponytail. Another helpful hint—if you're over seventeen, keep away from middle parts. They may look fine on teenagers, but just like other middle parts, they have a way of spreading with age. The best place to part hair is on the right side. Hair grows naturally from left to right; by parting it on the right you consistently comb against the natural growth which results in adding greater height and better fullness. Past a certain age, short hair seems to lift the lines of the face far better than does long hair. There comes a time when adopting teenage hairstyles is simply the worst move anyone can make.

If you want to get with it and are contemplating an Afro style, Rudel offers this timely news. Men and women are tiring of the full-blown Afro which, until recently, was the height of inness. As a result, Rudel has come up with a modified Afro, the "Afro shag." It's a longer look that befits the longer trend in today's female fashions. The cut lends itself nicely to many styles, is more natural, and is not as limiting as the original Afro. To successfully style the Afro shag, Rudel recommends styling be done on straight hair, cut approximately four inches long at the sides and the nape of the neck. Afro hair, he says, that has not been straightened often becomes problem hair as it has a tendency to break and must be combed through daily. On the other hand, straight hair is easier to manage; in fact, straightening can be good, especially if combined with monthly conditioning treatments. After the hair is straightened, it is shampooed and then set on small rods to create a curly Afro look. The curly set is easy to maintain and lasts a full two weeks. Anyone can learn to set the style at home. In Rudel's Afro department, where anyone can walk in and walk out wearing any Afro style, most choose the Afro shag, as opposed to the full-blown Afro, which received such rave notices in the past.

Summer Styling Hints

When summer comes along—be prepared. With a proper head start, heat and humidity need never hinder your style nor dampen your spirit. Start by analyzing past summertime hair problems. Does your usually nice, thick, straight, well-behaved hair fall apart under the combination of too much heat and humidity? Or do you have fine, straight hair that collapses at the first sign of summertime? Are you blessed with nice, wavy hair that expands to a matted mess of wispy strands as the air around you gets damper and hotter?

The extent to which you are affected by heat and humidity depends, again, on the texture and amount of hair you have. No matter whether your curly hair winds up in a mass of summertime frizzies or whether your hair is straight and falls to a limp flip-flop, you can control the situation by adopting the right hair style and using products made specifically for your type of hair.

For limp or fine hair that collapses at the first sign of humidity, try one of the new preparations made especially to combat high temperatures and humidity. For keeping your set together on hot humid days or nights, Dep's Small Wonder Styling Gel does the trick. Limp hair gets extra body with protein Conditioner Shampoo by Cosmetic Products of Ardsley; Clairol's Great Body, a real body-building conditioner, helps keep long, fine hair from falling into limp, stringy strands. Bio-Kur Extrahold Conditioner and Setting Formula works marvels to keep fine hair in place. Limp or fine hair set with Max Factor's Tried and True Hair Thickener stands up against the worst temperatures. To give you an aroma that is as nice as you look, try Chantilly Perfumed Hair Spray by Houbigant; it holds flyaway ends right where they belong.

For curly, coarse, or medium-textured hair that expands to a knotted mass of snarls or curls every time the temperature starts to soar, protect your style in advance by spraying lightly with Final Net Invisible Hair Spray by Ellen Kaye Cosmetics; Pantene's Treatment de Pantene also helps keep your hair under control, even when the humidity runs wild. L'Oréal's Conditioner and Setting Lotion with sunscreen protectors and protein additives gives sun-frazzled locks conditioning benefits, while setting hair where it belongs. Revlon's Flex Conditioner helps to tame expanded locks into neat, well-behaved hair.

Lastly, when the temperature starts to climb, adopt a style that won't disintegrate. Experiment with bound pigtails or a loosely pulled and colorfully bound ponytail. Try for a perky look with a double set of loose ponytails, tied neatly in ribbons behind each ear. Simple off-the-face styles will keep you looking fresh and appealing all summer long.

The Set

Skillful setting makes your style become a reality. It also makes the difference between cheers and tears. Fortunately, hair setting is an art anyone can learn. All it takes is know-how and faithful practice. A haircut will give your chosen style its contour, but it is the set that makes the style last from one shampoo to the next.

The basic necessities needed for setting your hair are setting lotion, rollers, hairpins, bobby pins, clips, and maybe cellophane tape. Lining up the right equipment makes the difference.

Modern setting lotions come in a variety of formulas designed to help thin, fine, or limp hair take on extra body. Searching for the lotion, gel, or spray that produces maximum holding results is well worth your while. Many of the latest products are packaged in small vials, with just enough liquid for one setting. Often they combine setting lotion and conditioning features. To find the best setting lotion, try buying several of the one-shot varieties until you find the one that gives your hair the body you need and want; the one that gives you instant bulk, and allows you to manage your hair from one shampoo till the next without any stickiness, dryness, or flimsiness. The use of beer as

Basic Hair-setting Equipment

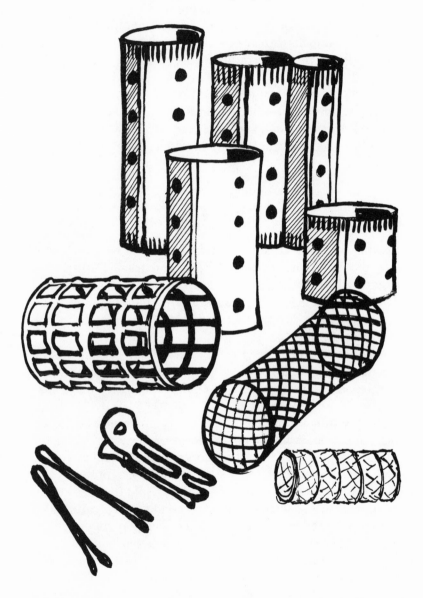

Four Standard Hair-setting Patterns

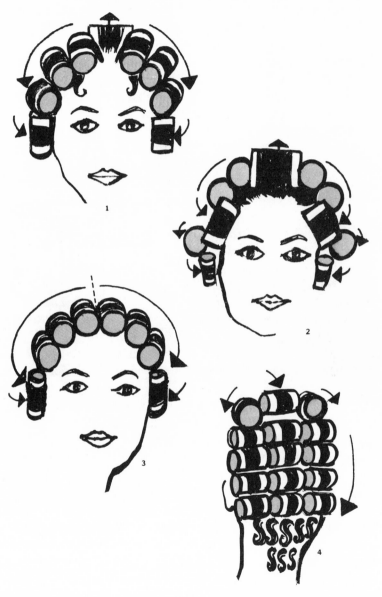

a setting lotion is not recommended, as most professionals find beer has a tendency to dry and dull hair. In emergencies, Knox Gelatin, or any other household brand, can be conjured into a setting lotion. Just dilute a spoonful of the granules in a glass of water. Under normal conditions if you really want to add body, try a product like Clairol's Great Body, or ask your salon about the Bodi-Endure treatment. It goes on like a shampoo and adds substance and texture that lasts up to six weeks. It also has a bonus effect in reducing the tangles which so often plague baby-fine hair.

Rollers, for styling height, width, or extra bulk and body, come in a variety of materials, diameters, designs, and lengths. Each type roller has its own special purpose. Small and medium rollers are especially useful for making curly, wavy, or sparse hair seem more abundant. Large and jumbo rollers give a smooth, sleek shape to virtually any hair style and are best suited for thick or coarse hair. A new ingenious pop-it kind of roller lets you adjust the size to suit your setting needs. To avoid splitting hair strands, eliminate any rollers which have teeth or sharp brushes in them.

Hair pins, bobby pins, and clips should never be older than one month, and should be rubber tipped and full of life and spring, if they are to offer maximum efficiency while protecting your hair and your set. Cellophane tape, too, developed specifically for hair needs, is a boon to hair setting. It can be used to secure curls and quiches on the cheeks or to hold bangs flat. It can even be threaded through curls as a substitute for the standard clip. Cellophane tape also has the advantage of holding your hair in place while you sleep, without poking your scalp as clips and bobby pins may.

To get set, start by combing a setting lotion evenly throughout the hair. Next, divide your hair into small sections for each hair roller. Begin at the back of the crown area. Take a lock of hair as wide and as thick as the roller. Hold the hair strand taut between your fingers. If your hair is tapered, the ends are broken, or if your hair is short, end-papers will help to achieve a smoother look for the finished product. Wrap an end-paper around the strand before winding. When rolling, hold the roller at a 45-degree angle from the scalp. Press hair ends—either enclosed in end-paper or without—around the roller, and wind evenly towards the scalp. There should be no pull on the roots. Rolling hair too tightly usually results in an aching scalp, or worse—damaged hair. Pulling hair too hard from the scalp creates too much tension and thus, as you roll, weak hairs are prone to snap and break off. Firm but easy tension is what it takes; it leaves room for shrinkage as the hair dries. To avoid leaving unwanted ridges, place your clips at the base of each roller, close to the scalp. As you roll your hair, try to envision the finished style and place your rollers accordingly.

To achieve firmer curl and more body, pin-curl the hair at the base of your set, in front of your ears and at the base of your neck. To wind a correctly shaped pin curl, start by picking up a strand of hair at the scalp; comb smooth; pull the hair in the direction in which the curl is to move; shape a round loop at the top of the hair and twist it around the end of your finger; slide the curled hair off your finger and clip the circled hair flat to the scalp. The more hair used in a pin curl, the looser the curl; less hair gives a tighter curl. To hold cheek pin curls in place, use one of the magic-cellophane hair tapes on the market.

You may want to try your hand at a finger curl. Finger curls are used for medium-to-long hair styles in place of rollers. To make this type of curl, wind a strand of hair around your finger almost as if your finger were a hair roller; slide your finger out of the curl; tuck the hair ends inside and pin in place. Stand-up curls can be used to create ringlets, spirals, or spaghetti curls. To make any one of these, start by combing a strand of hair straight out from the scalp; then, starting at the end of the strand, begin twisting the hair around the end of your finger until you have reached the scalp. Pull your finger out of the curl and clip the curl close to the scalp without flattening the curl.

Of the nonroller-type curls, the pin curl is used most often, as it makes the firmest curl. For extraneat pin curls without spring-away ends, be sure to tuck hair ends inside the circular curl before pinning in place. Clips are best for securing pin curls and other types of curls, as they leave no ridges on hair as bobby pins do.

Here, now, is a standard pattern for a basic set which can be combed out into a variety of smooth styles. Divide your hair into both a right and a left part, and wind three or four rollers backwards on the center hair from forehead to crown. Add four or five more rollers and continue rolling in a down-and-back direction from crown to the nape of the neck. Next to each side of the front hairline, wind two or three rollers downward to the ears; then move to the back and wind the remaining hair in a downward direction. Set hair at the very nape of the neck in pin curls. For cheek curls, wind two or three pin curls in front of each ear and tape. For a flipped-out look, try rolling the entire bottom row of curlers upward instead of down. For hair that is short, instead of continuing the rollers all the way to the nape of the neck, set the lower portion of hair in the back in pin curls.

If you prefer a curly look to a smooth look, part your hair in the center and wind the first roller parallel to the part in a downward direction; then wind a second and a third roller continuing in a downward path. Repeat the process on the other side of the part. Side rollers should also be wound downwards. Use small or medium-sized rollers to achieve the curly look you are after.

When hair has completely dried, comes the final stage—the all-important "comb out." Carefully remove rollers, pins, and papers. Avoid any hasty yanking, pulling, or tugging, so as not to break or tangle your hair. Next, rub a bit of hair cream on your hairbrush to add extra gloss; brush all of the hair back. Don't worry about taking out the curl; brushing blends roller separations and adds spring to your set. Brush your hair into the shape and contour of your style. If you want a pageboy look, make the hair turn under by combing or brushing your hair over your hand, keeping your hand close to the side of your head. If you want a flip, place your hand against the side of your head and comb your hair up and over your fingers.

If your style requires height or bulk, as most do, a little teasing may be needed. Teasing will help to give a longer-lasting line, but must be handled correctly and carefully or your hair may wind up a mass of tangles. Start by dividing your hair at the crown. Take a two-inch section of hair and hold it taut, straight up in the air. Next, with either a brush or nonmetal comb, very gently begin back-combing, starting at the roots and lightly combing downward to produce a slightly matted effect. Work from the scalp to about one-third of the way along the strand. Do not tease to the very ends of the strand. The idea is to try to create a foundation of teased hair close to scalp level over which the unteased hair can be smoothly draped and arranged. When finished teasing the crown, follow the same procedure; tease the side and back areas in the same manner. When your whole head is teased, pick up a small styling brush and lightly reshape your hair into the contour which your style requires. If hair becomes knotted or tangled as you brush it out, the hair has been overteased. Teasing should last twenty-four hours and should be brushed out at the end of the day.

A word of warning—if you hairdresser has told you not to tease your hair, follow his advice and choose a style that does not require back-combing. When brushing teased hair, brush only the surface layers; if the bristles of your brush penetrate the top layer of hair, you may brush out the foundation you have just created. Begin by styling the crown area first; then move to the sides. Leave the front for last. Don't be afraid to use your fingers as well as your brush to create and sculpt your style. To curb problem strands that spring up, apply a film of hairdressing to the palms of your hands and pat your hair gently. You can control a droopy strand by turning it into a tight pin curl. Tuck the curl underneath the outer layer or keep it in place with a decorative clip. For hairs that pop out of place, put hair spray on your comb and skim hair lightly. When you have achieved the perfect look, spray your hairdo lightly to preserve it. At this point you may want to add a groovy or glittering touch; jewelry for the hair can serve decorative as well as practical purposes. Headbands, barrettes, combs, or ribbons all help keep hair in place while adding a personal flair. There are endless accents through which you can reveal your personality. Beads, leather, bows, or rhinestones are all indications of you and your personality.

17.
Straightening and Waving –
The Pros and Cons

"It's enough to make your hair curl" doesn't have to be just a cute saying. Today's modern permanenting products make it possible to achieve just the amount of curl you want whether it be maximum curl, a little wave, or an out-of-sight curve.

Hair-permanenting techniques and products have come a long way since 1939 when the cold wave was first introduced. In those days permanenting was almost tantamount to torture. If the grip of the curlers didn't get you, the odor itself was bound to be overpowering. Today's salon and home products make permanenting a simple, painless, almost pleasurable procedure.

First, the hair must be shampooed to remove any accumulated oil, grease, or hair spray; then a chemical solution is distributed through the hair. The solution remains on the hair for two to twenty minutes, based on the formula and the manufacturer's instructions. After the proper length of time has elapsed, the hair is wound around plastic curlers to urge it into its new shapely, curly contour. For natural-looking curls, the largest rollers provided should be used. The smaller the rollers, the tighter the curls will turn out. Merely to keep hair in line without real curls, there are body waves which use overall large curling rods to give hair more substance. After the prescribed time has passed the hair is rinsed with a neutralizing agent to rid it of the chemicals used to promote the curl or body. Permanents remain permanent for anywhere from three to six months depending upon the hair's texture.

Visiting a salon equipped with experienced operators proficient in the art of permanent waving ensures that your hair will be analyzed for texture and condition so that the proper type and strength of permanent will be prescribed.

If you wish to go it alone, you can. Today's modern home-permanent products are specifically labled for all hair types—fine, coarse, soft, or normal. Current permanenting products, whether they be home or salon types, all contain special conditioning agents which restore natural oils just as quickly as they are removed by waving chemicals. Damage from chemicals is, therefore, almost nil. Most damage, when and if it occurs, is the result of winding the hair too tightly on the permanenting curlers. Damage results not only because of excess tension but also because the waving lotion and the neutralizer are not able to circulate freely through each of the hair strands. If handled properly and timed correctly today's permanents are not harmful. It is important, however, to follow the explicit timing recommendations given by the manufacturer.

Never wave over already permanented hair. Never use metallic brush rollers, metal bobby pins, or clips with any permanent-wave solution; the chemical reaction to metal is extremely hazardous. If end-papers are specified and included, use them. Always start with a preview test curl before proceeding further. This is especially important for bleached or dyed hair. Since certain individuals experience negative skin reactions to permanent-waving chemicals, just as others may react negatively to tomatoes or penicillin, a preview test curl should be tried by anyone who is planning to have a permanent wave. If an allergy is evident, stop there. Give in to nature and resign yourself to

The Wrap-around System: Hair Straightening Without the Use of Chemicals

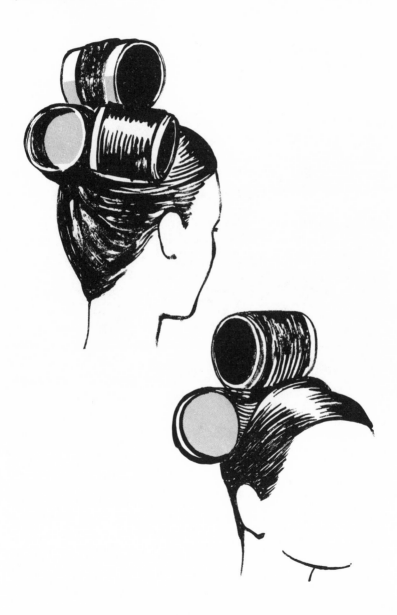

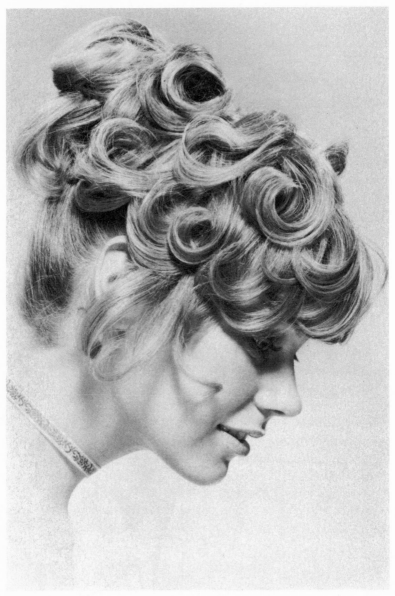

Modern permanent products make it possible to achieve just the amount of curl you want. Courtesy of Clairol Inc.

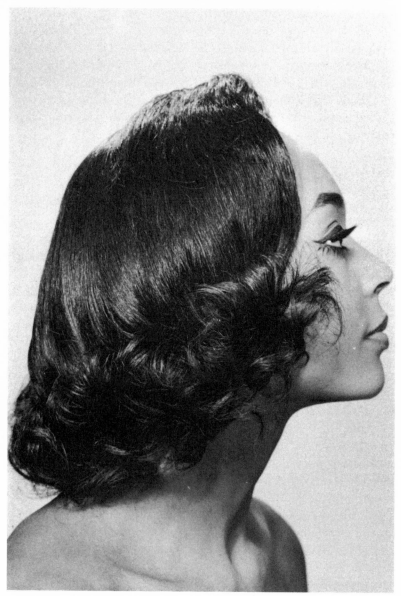

*Chemical hair-straightening is really a permanent in reverse.
Courtesy of Calirol Inc.*

the fact that your hair was not intended to be curly. Find an alternate style that does not call for permanenting.

One well-known New York hairdresser, before proceeding with permanenting or hair coloring, makes it a point to ask whether the customer's menstrual period is due within the next three days. If the answer is affirmative, the appointment is rescheduled for the following week. It is his firm conviction that glandular changes during this time doom the success of hair coloring and permanent waving.

Straightening

Chemical straightening is really a permanent in reverse. It's not a temporary arrangement; once it's straight, it's straight and that's it, unless you cut it off. Although home-curl-relaxer kits are sold over the counter, the process of hair straightening is best left to the able hands of an expert. Even though straightening chemicals are akin to those used in permanenting, overall straightening is a considerably harsher form of treatment.

Unlike permanenting, where you wind hair into curls, once the hair has been chemically saturated and commanded into submission, it is combed out straight and then subsequently rehardened with a neutralizer. Straightening hair requires expert care and lots of conditioning.

Hair straightening is one of the few beauty operations for which many salons require a signed customer release before any work whatsoever is begun; this is due to the built-in hazards. Fine, kinky hair does not always respond well to straightening. Even without experiencing any hair loss, hair may suddenly appear scant and limp. Dyed hair should never be straightened, as the combination of chemicals can easily lead to hair breakage at scalp level, therby leaving bald areas in sight. Inept operators are few and far between; nevertheless, it is important to shop carefully for a reputable salon. Check out various salons where friends have had work done, know in advance whether a release is, or is not, required. Straightening should be done as infrequently as possible; in general, no more often than twice a year. Harsh chemicals and too much processing can easily cause permanent damage to hair follicles. Unless there is no alternative, it is wisest to avoid chemical straightening.

George Michael, king of the long-hairs, also straightens without chemicals. His technique is to retrain hair and, though it may take up to two years, followers of his system are with him every step of the way.

New York stylist Louis Gignac also swears that he can make the kinkiest hair shiny and straight without use of chemicals. His technique is a wrap-around system of repeated brushing and winding of wet hair that wraps itself around the head and sets itself straight. His technique is a simple one; the head is utilized as one giant hair roller. To add extra height, Louis adds three extralarge rollers at the crown. Working with clean, wet hair, he places the three rollers on top and proceeds to section the hair, combing each section over the forehead and around the head, clipping the ends temporarily in place. He continues to part, section, and wrap in one direction. Clips are removed as the wrapping progresses so that no ridges will occur. Then endpapers soaked in setting lotion are plastered over the head to keep flyaway ends in place. A hair net adds extra protection. Then it's under the hair dryer until the hair is absolutely dry. Louis's own wrap-around kit—three large rollers, setting lotion in a spray bottle, end-papers, rattail comb, clips, hair net, and instruction sheet—are sold by mail. The cost $7, tax and postage included. (Louis-Guy D', 12 East 57th Street, New York City 10022.)

Ironing hair as a method of hair straightening is a technique which is vetoed by every expert. The reasons are fairly obvious—besides being an inefficient means of straightening, the chances of hair breakage by scorching are enormous. Leave your flat iron to the job for which it was built, that of pressing clothes, not your hair.

If your hair is too curly for your taste, you can have it straightened professionally or you can use one of the home hair-straightening kits on the market. Before using a product, be sure to read the manufacturer's directions and make a strand test to determine just how long the straightening lotion should be left on the hair in order to achieve the desired results. An initial strand test and proper timing are absolutely necessary to ensure favorable results.

Electrical Devices

A home hair dryer beats a turkish towel for hair drying purposes every time. It also means that a shampoo and set can be accomplished in about an hour's time. If it's just a matter of a few curls, they can be restored in minutes. On top of other benefits, a set dried speedily under a dryer outlasts a set which is allowed to dry naturally. There are several dryers now on the market that are steam-emitting models. Utilizing this type, you can roll up your hair dry between shampoos and, because of the moisture influence, wind up with an almost good-as-new set.

Electric curlers are the latest, newest, and nicest things to happen to hair setting in a long time. Now you can switch your hair style almost as easily as your mood. All it takes is ten minutes. Instant hair setters give your hair the pzzazz it needs for extra body and great, long-lasting styling.

There are two varieties of electric hair-setting units on the market, a dry and a steam type. Costs for either one vary between $10 and $50 depending on the brand name and the number of added goodies included (extra curlers, special setting lotion, head cap, etc.).

Instant hair setters all work along the same lines—even such elaborate sets as Lady Schick, Remington Steam Rollers, and the Kindness Custom-Care Setter by Clairol. First, the unit is plugged in so that the rollers automatically heat up on individual heating posts. When the red dots on the rollers turn nearly black, the rollers are ready for use. It takes roughly ten minutes for the rollers to reach their controlled degree of

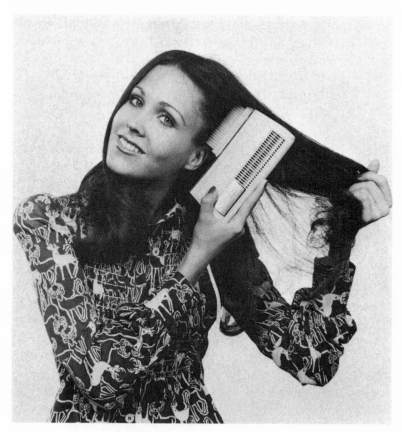

The electric air brush styling dryer is one of today's electrical hair styling devices. Courtesy of Clairol Inc.

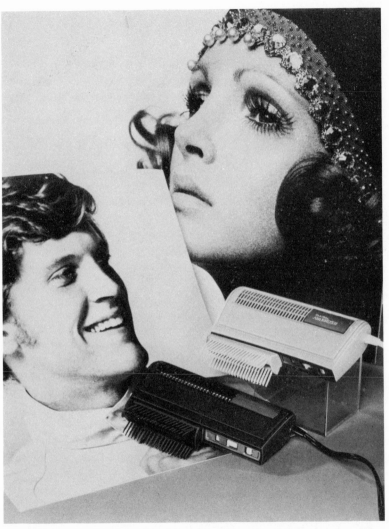

*It's a his-and-her hair world, a new era in hair care freedom.
Courtesy of Clairol Inc.*

Today's Electrical Hair-helping Devices

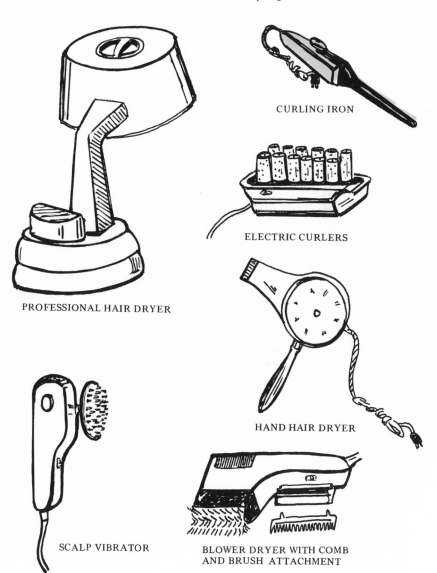

CURLING IRON

ELECTRIC CURLERS

PROFESSIONAL HAIR DRYER

HAND HAIR DRYER

SCALP VIBRATOR

BLOWER DRYER WITH COMB
AND BRUSH ATTACHMENT

warmth. As one roller is removed from its post, a fresh roller should be placed on the empty post. By following this rotation, you are sure of having enough hot rollers to use if your head requires extra curlers. Theoretically, by the time you place the last roller in your hair, the first fresh roller will be ready, in case it is needed.

At no time should heated electric dry rollers be left in the hair for more than ten minutes. Any form of excessive heat applied directly to the hair over a long period will either dry or scorch hair. Unlike dry rollers, steam rollers remain in the hair until they are cool, which requires at least 15 minutes. When removing the rollers, take care not to tangle or pull the curls. After the hair has cooled sufficiently, just comb and style. It's as easy as rolling off a log.

Just one final reminder—electric hair curlers are a marvel for last-minute special occasions; however, they are not recommended as an everyday curling method. Constant use may result in loss of hair. Every time you pull out a roller, a hair or two gets left behind in its teeth. Needless to say, with constant and continual use, the number of lost hairs multiplies. Excessive heat can easily disintegrate the hair or leave it dry and brittle, easily susceptible to breakage. When they are reserved for special use, however, there is no great loss and, for this reason alone, electric curlers are important.

The rise in popularity of the instant hair setter has paved the way for numerous new products designed to accompany the instant hair setter. They are offered primarily to combat possible drying effects caused by overheating. Most are aimed at conditioning the hair while adding extra-hold benefits. Among the latest newcomers are Dippity-Do Heated Roller Condition Set; Kindness Heat Activated Conditioner, a protein-enriched liquid to replace ordinary steam with a penetrating conditioning mist which sets and beautifies in one step without leaving hair gummy, sticky, or dry; Remington Hair Conditioner, made to be used in conjunction with Lady Remington steam rollers, and promises a longer lasting set—up to twenty-four hours—along with super conditioning benefits; Dep's Plugged In, a spray setting lotion, which claims to make electric curls last up to three and four times longer as well as protecting hair from becoming dry or split—all you do is spray and roll, for a set that holds and holds.

Instant setters and their accompanying conditioning products can be used on all types of hair—dyed, tinted, permanented, or straightened. The curling action of instant setters is so brief and so efficient that there isn't normally time for heat damage to occur to hair. Handling of hot curlers can however, result in the accidental burning of fingers. Before winding the first hot roller, protect your fingers from burns and blisters by applying a plastic bandage over the tip of each thumb and index finger. Properly handled instant setters offer the advantage of doing away with sleeping on rollers or killing time sitting under a hair dryer. By comparison, they make the old, electric curling iron seem antiquated.

If you still own an *electric curling iron,* though, hang on to it. It may not make an ideal hair-setting implement, but it is a good styling tool, provided heat is not applied for any excessive period; a few seconds per curl is all you need. The main advantage of a curling iron is you can put curls exactly where you want them and make them just as curly as you want. Quick ringlets, fluffy loose curls, or tight masses of curls can all be conjured up with a twist of the wrist.

A curling iron also allows you to restore style to a flip, fluff, or any deflated do—or, conversely, even relax curls that are too curly. If rather than remove waves you want to add tight curls, start by selecting a small hair strand, pull the curling iron through the strand, clamp the hair in place and lock the roller, twirl the curling iron and hold in position for a moment or two. After a few seconds, pull the iron out.

Variations include sweeping your hair up, pinning it in place, and creating lots of tight little curls on top—or, if you prefer, try making dangling ringlets using your curling iron.

A small word of caution—since home curling irons are not generally thermostatically controlled, it is best to underheat them so as not to risk singeing hair. Never use a curling iron on hair that has been chemically straightened or it will most certainly result in hair breakage. Use of this technique on bleached or permanented hair is also to be avoided, as it is likely to damage hair.

The *electric, hand hair dryer* is another of today's electrical devices at your disposal. Anyone who has ever seen a professional at work knows that a hand hair dryer can be a very useful styling implement, if you know how to use it. So, here's how. First, with a brush in one hand and the electric hand dryer—or blower, as it is sometimes called—in the other, brush a lock of wet hair in the shape and direction you want. By directing *warm* air from the blower onto the shaped lock, the curl is dried and set in place. By jetting air up and under the hair, you can add extra fullness to your hair and give your style a nice, well-rounded contour. Applying a light spray of hair-setting liquid or gel before using the blower will give your style lasting beauty.

With a hand hair dryer, heat should never be directed right up against the scalp, since there is danger of scorching hair and scalp. On the "high" set, blower heat reaches infernal intensity. Do not play with this sort of fire at close range or you will be burned. Singed hair or a burnt scalp can be avoided by maintaining moderate heat and a generous distance between the blower and your scalp.

There's also the *electric brush* or the *electric comb* or a combination. Brush and comb attachments fit neatly into a hand-blower apparatus which allows for simultaneous styling and drying without danger of singeing. This all-in-one unit helps you to get the swinging natural look professionals achieve. Many units come with a wide-comb attachment to help create an overall shape, plus a narrow comb for handling styling details, plus a brush to provide bulk and fullness. An electric brush dries faster than a standard hand blower.

For feminine beauty, there is the new Lady Schick Air Styler; for men there is the new Schick Styling Dryer. Solis, a professional blower from Switzerland, favored by many Los Angeles pros, can be found in beauty supply shops for about

$20. The Hot Comb by Remington also helps a fellow tackle his cowlick problems while keeping his long-styled hair from looking out of place. The Clairol Air Brush styling dryers—his and hers—usher in a new era of hair-care freedom for everybody who wants great-looking, now hair. Men also have the Current Comb at their disposal. It styles, waves, or straightens, heats instantly and includes a power-handle styling comb-and-brush attachment, all for $15. Available through Hair Imports of Colorado Springs, Colorado.

Other miscellaneous electrical hair appliances include the electrical heating cap and the electric scalp vibrator or massager. The Wella heat cap, generally available for purchase through beauty supply houses, is designed for use with a conditioner whose beneficial effects are enhanced by the use of the heat cap.

As far as the electric scalp massager is concerned, just plug it in and your scalp tingles with excitement. Used faithfully, a vibrator helps to relieve the tensions which many professionals attribute to loss of hair. It also aids in improving scalp circulation by bringing better blood nutrition to hair roots. On top of these benefits, it helps to distribute scalp oils.

Anyone who is seriously bothered by falling hair or dandruff can fight back vigorously with use of a scalp vibrator. The cost usually runs between $8 and $12.

18.
Women's Hairpieces –
Natural Vs. Synthetic, Man-Made Vs. Machine-Made

Wigs work wonders; it's no wonder, then, that they have gone to the heads of millions of smart women. For virtually every hair problem a wig supplies a solution.

Take the case of Miss Kilpatrick, a fourth-grade teacher, pretty, popular, self-assured, and about as bald as the globe of the world sitting on her desk. (This last fact she managed to keep smartly concealed from students and friends alike.) Miss Kilpatrick had not always been bald. A year earlier, she had had her own crop of pretty red hair, styled almost in the same way as the wig she now wore. One morning she awoke to find small clumps of hair on her pillow. As she frantically ran her hands over her head, to her shock, she discovered several bare circular areas on her scalp. Immediately, she rushed to her doctor's office and that afternoon her physician diagnosed her hair loss as alopecia areata, a perplexing form of baldness. Although she was informed that, in most cases the condition does not worsen, in Miss Kilpatrick's case hair continued to fall until not a hair remained.

Wigs, while giving Miss Kilpatrick and others like herself cosmetic relief, also provide an enormous emotional lift. For those suffering from thinning hair, temporary hair loss after childbirth, falling hair following illness, high fever, drug reaction, mental trauma, or a rundown condition, wigs offer the wearer a tremendous morale boost while the course of treatment continues.

Wigs are marvelous, too, for the long-hair types who love short hair, but can't stand the thought of cutting it off. For those who want to let their own hair grow but don't have the patience to wait for the miracle to happen, a wig works more instantaneous magic. When your hairdo goes haywire, pop on a wig and you're all together again. On special occasions that call for last-minute glamour and sophistication, especially for the busy working girl, a hairpiece is the answer to a maiden's prayers. Convenience, variety, fun, and cutting down on beauty-parlor visits are extra incentives for owning a wig, in addition to the practical advantages of giving hair a rest from constant exposure, setting, teasing, permanent waving, bleaching, or tinting. Whether one wears a wig out of necessity or for pure pleasure, women have every reason under the sun to love their store-bought tresses.

No longer are hairpieces the favorite topic of vaudeville comedians; the stigma of wearing a wig is definitely part of history. Today, estimated wig sales total approximately $500 million. With an approximate 8.5 million women wearing hairpieces, this means that one out of every four women owns one wig or more. The deceivers are everywhere in a multitude of forms; so no matter which you now own or are planning to buy, be sure to call it by its correct name.

Wigs

A wig is a full-sized hairpiece which covers the entire hair-growth area of the head. Wigs can be long, short, or medium, with or without a part. Besides being any length, they can be just about any color.

Selections from the Leon Amendola Collection of Hair Pieces

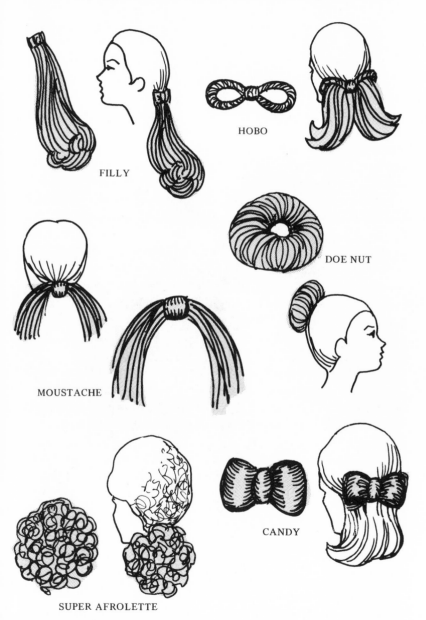

FILLY

HOBO

DOE NUT

MOUSTACHE

SUPER AFROLETTE

CANDY

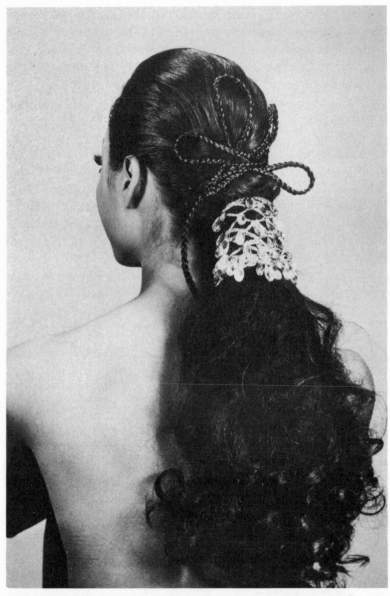

Switch: a long piece of hair fastened at one end. Can be knotted, braided or ponytailed. Courtesy of Clairol Inc.

Wiglets

A wiglet is a small hairpiece worn to blend in with your natural hair and is generally used to add height to the top of the head. It can also act as an excellent cover-up for thinning hair. Wiglets, both big and little, cover any area of the head and come in several forms—either as one curl, a cluster of curls, or as a straight, hanging-loose shock. This variety of hairpiece leads all others in sales.

Falls

A fall is a small piece with either straight or curly hair which falls from the crown of the head to shoulder length or even longer. A fall helps to give hair extra fullness and added shape.

Switches

A switch is a long piece of hair fastened at one end; it can be knotted, beaded, braided, pony-tailed, or twisted into a variety of forms such as a chignon, a bun, or it may be intertwined with the wearer's own hair.

Cascades

A cascade is a cluster of hair on a long, narrowed, tapered base. It is generally worn in long curls which fall down the back or sides.

Pin-On-Curls

Individual curls or a small group of curls on a miniature base which can be pinned onto the natural hair or added to a hairpiece are called pin-on-curls. Those of contrasting color are referred to as frosting rings.

Bangs

A row of short hair strands which covers the forhead and can be attached under a hairpiece or blended into the natural hairline are called bangs, which is what they are.

Variations

Other ingenious creations, as exemplified by the Leon A-mendola collection, include such fascinating nomenclature as Filly, Hobo, Moustache, Moustache Bow, etc. (See sketches for full details.)

Selecting a Wig

The wig you purchase should fit comfortably. If the band surrounding the wig is too small, don't rely on its stretching. More than likely, it will painfully pop off your head just when you least expect it to. If the band is too large, you can have a hairdresser correct it for you, or you can do it yourself by taking a tuck in the band and sewing down the rim. The wig you are considering should follow your hairline and should cover the nape of your neck. If the wig is too short in the back, you won't fool anyone. Besides fitting correctly, it should have swing and movement, too. If your wig is too heavy, you're bound to look wiggy and artificial. Consider your facial structure. Is it oval, heart-shaped, round, square? Follow the same guide lines recommended for styling. Wigs, too, can minimize weaknesses and play up positive features. Avoid selecting a wig which is far from your own natural hair color, or your skin tones may not blend well with it. If you do make a radical color change, chances are that your makeup will also need to change radically. Duplicating your own hair color exactly may be difficult. Matching must be done in good light, or later it may come to light that the wig you have selected has too much red highlight in it. A good match can be assured if you color your hair to match the hairpiece.

The choice is yours—a full wig for all-over cover-up, a fall for extra fullness, a wiglet for top curls, or a switch for variety. You get what you pay for so, before you invest, be sure to have all the facts.

Natural Hair Versus Synthetics

Hairpieces made from human hair are considered tops in quality, due to their credibility. Virgin hair—undamaged by coloring, bleaching, or permanent waving—is superior to tampered hair. Nowadays, virgin hair is a rarity and, therefore, it is expensive. The label "Real Hair" does not automatically mean *human* hair. In a cheap wig, it could very well be horse, dog, or monkey hair. "Real Hair" in white or silver wigs might be angora, sheep, yak, or vicuna.

Wigs constructed of human hair have differing grades. European hair is considered the most desirable, because it comes in a wide range of colors and has good elasticity. Sometimes, however, European hair is blended with Oriental or Asian hair, so that a label "100-percent Human Hair, European Made" does not necessarily mean 100-percent European hair. American hair is not considered up to par with European tresses, as very often it has been colored, bleached, or permanented. Even though American hair may not be considered the very tops, here's an idea. If you are having your own mane cut off, don't sweep away the lost locks. Use them to make your own pin-on curls; just cover the top inch of the curls with a strong clear-drying glue and a few wraps of thread. When dry, set and pin on. Generally speaking, American hair is rarely used in hairpieces. The source of top quality wigs belongs to our

European cousins. Differentiating by nationality, experts agree that Italian hair—the very best-textured (medium fine)—holds a set well, has a nice silky feel, and looks sumptuously luxurious. French hair, also fine-textured and silky, does not hold a set quite as well, and under pressure of humidity tends to fall limp. Spanish hair, medium coarse in texture, has good lustre, but feels less silky. It usually retains a set well. Conclusion: if you're seeking curls, look into an Italian-or Spanish-hair wig for best quality.

Gray, light pale, and auburn hair are distinguished as extra colors and command higher prices than the more common shades. Color is not limited to any one particular country. Light-colored hair frequently is obtained from Germany and Austria. Darker shades very often are obtained from the south of France. In southern France, the cultivation and sale of hair by peasant girls is a common practice. Fairs are held for the explicit purpose of selling hair to merchants for ultimate use in wigs.

The Orient is another prime source of wig hair. Oriental wigs are less expensive than their European counterparts. The very best oriental hair comes from Japan, Indonesia, China, and Korea. Indonesian women, too, are helping increase the family budget by cutting off their lovely knee-length hair to sell to hair merchants. The demand for hair from Indonesia is so great that robbers have been known to cut off the hair of women riding in crowded Djakarta busses.

Oriental hair is strong, but very often coarser and more difficult to curl than European hair; quality and color range is more limited. In general, Asian hair is coarse-textured, glossy, naturally straight and, therefore, tends to reject curly setting. If you are looking for a simple, sleek wig, however, it is well worth investigating.

What's in a name? Everything, when it comes to synthetic wigs. "Dolly M," "Delilah," "Maria," "Monique," "Suzanne," "Audrey," "Rebecca," "Veronica," "Heidi," "Gilda," "Martinique," "Gaucho," "Gypsy," "Shag," "Veil," "Vagabond," "Phaedra," "Marguerite," "Cheryl," "Samantha," "Noel," "April," "Eve," "Tami," "Mad-Mad," as well as many more, all aptly named and styled to transform you into all the people you are or ever dreamed of being. Although the first man-made synthetic fibers used in hairpieces lacked the naturalness and durability of human hair, today's synthetics cost less than hair wigs and require practically no care. They are permanently curled and completely washable. Because of tapered back styling and a stretch base, they fit almost every size head with comfort. Names in synthetic fibers include: Dynel, Polemer Spun Hair, Kankelon, Emrelon (a European synthetic), Monsanto's new modacrylic Elura fiber, and Chatellon's Venicelon, which claims such realism that it takes a chemist to tell the difference between it and beautiful, healthy hair. The makers boast that Venicelon fibers are round like human hair, textured like fine Italian hair, and can be curled, restyled, sprayed, and even shampooed back to an original style. For little more than a song, you can own a synthetic wig, fall, or wiglet, just perfect to toss on after swimming, for an impromptu night out, or for the most elegant of affairs. No matter where you sport your hairpiece, you can go in confidence. The synthetic pretenders are all so realistic and easy to care for that surely Mother Nature must suddenly feel just a bit sheepish.

Man-Made Versus Machine-Made

How a wig is processed is perhaps even more important than the type of hair of which it is composed. Wigs are either hand-tied or machine-sewn. Hand-tied wigs are lighter than machine-made wigs. Each hair of a hand-tied wig is double knotted into a mesh foundation. The tighter the knot, the less likely it is to be brushed away. The individual hairs are hand-sewn in the direction in which hair naturally grows. This is important for appearance's sake and manageability. One of the reasons custom-made European wigs are costly is that it takes a wig craftsman at least a week to turn out a hand-tied wig, but the workmanship never fails.

In a machine-made wig, strands are attached to the base by a sewing machine. In general, machine-made wig caps are firmer and hold their shape better than hand-made wigs because the hairs are sewn in circular rows. Instead of fastening one to five strands as is done in constructing a hand-made wig, machines clump together as many as thirty hairs or fibers, sometimes leaving open areas on either side of a multistrand grouping—this leading, unfortunately, to less manageability. Machine-made synthetic wigs have, however, been refined to the nth degree and are excellent pretenders. Oriental wigs are most often machine-made. Some are constructed "half and half," as are many of the European wigs. In this type of construction, the back of the hairpiece is machine-made, and the front is hand-tied. Hand-finished edges add a very natural-looking hairline; they cost less than hand-made wigs and very often look equally good. The conclusion—a hand-made wig will, in the long run, offer better durability and stay in the best of shape, but the difference in price between man-made versus a machine-made wig may seem incredible. Bear in mind, though, that there are wigs for just about every pocketbook. Although a virgin, custom-made, dyed wig costs about $300, a first-quality human-hair machine-made wig can be had for about $50. It's possible to get good-looking wigs, falls, and cascades for as little as $17; wiglets for half as much. The thing to do is to decide what you need and how much you want to spend, then consult a reputable shop.

Good-looking low-cost hairpieces with a money-back guarantee are also offered nationally via mail order. A word of caution—be aware of extra-special good deals or unrealistic prices. There are get-rich swindlers even in the wig market!

With these facts stashed beneath your cap, calculating what's best for you should be far easier.

Proper Wearing

Putting a hairpiece on doesn't mean plunking it down. With the proper know-how, it's possible to stash nearly any length, width, or breadth of hair beneath a wig. Furthermore, with the right technique, there's no chance that your natural hair will be harmed, unless the method of attachment produces excessive pulling on the scalp. To avoid unnecessary problems, here's the right way of getting it on. Begin by brushing all of your own hair back; then pull all of the hair to one side and run a line of bobby pins up the back of your head. French-twist the hair, so it lies flat in the back by bringing the ends up and winding in a wide circle on top of your crown. This helps to distribute the hair evenly. When getting your head into the wig, be sure that the wig is centered properly so that its contour coincides with your own real hairline. Although wigs even come equipped with a fastening comb, for extra security you may want to anchor the wig again with a few unseen bobby pins. Check to be certain that the wig comb is inserted without causing undue scalp tension. In the case of a stretch wig, anchoring presents no problems since stretchables usually fit as neatly as a bathing cap—except they're a lot cooler.

If you've been delaying under the illusion that wig-wearing may cause hidden damage to your own real hair, relax. More often wig-wearing spells salvation. While wigging out, damaged home-grown hair gets the time it needs to grow out unnoticed, without further exposure to dye, bleach, hair straightening, or permanenting. Experts, nevertheless, remind the wig wearers that its healthy for the scalp to "breath" some of the time, so don't wear out your wig morning, noon, and night. When you're home alone, take it off and do refrain from wearing it while you sleep. The time to put it on is when you're going out.

Falls

To be 100 percent credible, a fall must be correctly placed. Some wearers, unfortunately, never seem to get the hang of it. They continually aim for a bump-at-the-back-of-the-head look with a too-rounded base, or a too-far-back placement. Once you have properly positioned your fall, securing it is easy, since most falls come with their own comb, which securely tucks right into the real hair. Sometimes the hang-up is the obvious line of demarcation between the real you and your fall. You can overcome this problem easily by simply working your own hair over the fall. Using a headband as cover up is also possible, but it's usually a dead giveaway. Don't let a headband be your downfall. Although using your own hair as a cover-up may take more time to arrange, the look is definitely more natural.

Wigs

As for wiglets, any wiglet can be made to look like it is a part of you, if you blend it with your own hair. You can hide where your hair ends and where the wiglet takes over by intertwining natural and fake curls together. For wiglets which are long hair (usually a twirl of curls), drape the ends over, around, and in with the ends of your own pinned-up hair. This way, every single strand looks like it belongs to you. Wiglets don't usually wiggle because they come with combs around the base. For extra security, pin a large pin curl or two under the wiglet and thread several large hairpins through the foundation into the pin curls. This way, your hairdo will stay put, no matter what.

The Top Names

If you don't own a hairpiece but plan to buy one, knowing the top names in today's ever-growing synthetic market is essential. When shopping, keep in mind the names of the following designers:

Givenchy—his beautiful wash-and-wear Dynel creations are renowned for their versatility, simplicity of care, and their complete natural look which is achieved through a hand-knotting technique. Designs such as Vagabond, Suzanne, and Audrey, his latest inspired by and named for actress/client Audrey Hepburn, can be combed and worn in varying styles, just like real hair. Givenchy wigs come in thirty-six colors, including sunstreaks.

Donald Brooks—creates in Dynel. Brooks' wigs often feature hand-tied construction combined with a brand-new process called Omniflex, which makes precurled fibers stand up from the wig foundation to simulate the way hair grows naturally from the scalp. Fibers can be brushed, combed, and even teased, just like your own hair.

Schiaparelli—this lovely lady creates her magic with Elura, Monsanto's modacrylic fibers. Schiaparelli-styled wigs have a natural sheen and are truly versatile. They can be wet and set, restyled; even heat doesn't harm Elura wigs. You can actually use electric rollers safely. Schiaparelli styles are available in twenty-one colors, including frosteds.

Lupe—this Cuban hairdresser, whose regular clientele includes notables like Mrs. William F. Buckley and sugar heiress Mrs. Andrew Fuller, is a newcomer to the field of commercial wig designing. Creating in Elura, his first three designs include a medium-long, versatile pageboy and two layered cuts: one long, the other short and touseled.

Jacque Kouri—a specialist in the styling and designing of women's wigs and falls who is known, however, to be equally adept in the handling of male hairpieces. In addition to his regular Park Avenue clientele, Arlene Frances and a well-known White House celebrity are said to be among his most devoted customers.

Wig Maintenance

Whether made of human hair or from one of the new synthetics, your wig requires care to survive gracefully. The normal life span of a reputable wig ranges from five to ten years, depending upon the care it is given.

The first step is to buy it a wig block. Wig blocks come in head sizes, like hat sizes (21″, 22″, 23″). Besides keeping your wig in good shape when not being worn, a wig block is an ideal support for setting your wig. Show that you really care by keeping your wig block in a cool area—avoid radiators or any other hot spots. When not in use, protect your hairpiece from dust and light by covering it with a silky scraf. To keep it really out of sight and free from dust, invest in a wig box, the handy carrying kind that has its own build-in block. You can't go wrong with this equipment.

The second step for top-notch maintenance is a proper cleansing agent. There are different uses for different wigs. For real hair, a good wig shampoo like Helene Curtis Wig Wash works effectively and safely. Following directions, pour enough liquid into a bowl to saturate the hairpiece. Dip the wig into the solution, hair-side down. Swish a few times, then gently squeeze the piece so that fluid moistens every hair and gets through to the backing. Rinse in clear water. To remove excess liquid, press between two towels; then blot dry several times. Place the wig back on its block. If hair strands appear excessively tangled or dull, use a good conditioning spray to add instant shine and manageability. Helene Curtis does it again with her wig conditioner. Let the wig dry for at least one hour before setting.

For human hairpieces, dry cleaning fluids work best. Dry cleaners contain no water and do not require diluting. Custom wig pieces call for dry cleaning because hand-tied knots loosen up in water. Dry-cleaning fluids are easy to use. Just dip a brush into the fluid and then run it gently through the hair. Wipe off excess with a towel and dry by fluffing hair with fingers or a comb. Although dry cleaning a wig is in itself a simple process, peripheral complications do exist. The agents found in dry cleaning fluids are derived from petroleum and have the same flammable characteristics as alcohol. Never clean a wig near an open flame. Do not smoke. Avoid using electrical appliances, gas heaters or any other device which produces flame or high heat during wig cleaning. To avoid sensitive reactions, should hands or even a table top be exposed to the fluid, wash them at once. Since dry cleaning fumes are pungent and, if inhaled, noxious, for your own safety clean your wig in a well ventilated room. Note that the pungent odor will disappear as soon as the wig is dry. Vapon Shampoo is an excellent dry cleaning fluid and is harmless when safety directions are followed. Style now puts out a nonflammable dry cleaning spray for human hair wigs.

To freshen up wigs between cleanings, there are instant dry cleaners. These come in spray form and can be used on honest-to-goodness hair or synthetics. Wig and Wiglet Cleaner by Tresses Unlimited and Helene Curtis' Instant Wig Cleaner both work efficiently in a matter of seconds. Just spray lightly and brush downward. If necessary, repeat again, starting at the top and working down. Let dry at room temperature.

If your life savings have gone to your head, you may be reluctant to douse your wig in any kind of liquid. Under the circumstances, the best solution for you is professional cleaning. Salon charges for cleaning and restyling run from $7.50 up for a small piece to $10 for a full wig.

To keep your wig in proper style requires gentle handling and careful setting. Remember, wig hairs don't grow back. The comb you use should ahve teeth spaced wide enough apart to untangle hair without pulling out precious strands. If you use a brush, be sure it's one designed especially for wigs. Setting lotions are off-limits for wigs as they thicken hair to the point that combing requires yanking which automatically means loss of valuable hairs.

For long-lasting beauty, professionals consistently stress the importance of a good first setting. Before beginning your set, make sure the wig is securely anchored to its block. For holding purposes T-pins are best, as the top cross bar acts as an anchor without tearing the wig's mesh foundation. With the wig securely in position, dampen its hair lightly with warm water and set just as you would your natural hair. Any type of roller can be used with one exception—brush rollers, which have a tendency to pull and catch at hairs. (They're not good for your own hair either!) When finished setting, leave the piece on its block and tie a net over it. Let it dry at room temperature. If you use a home dryer, place it on a cool setting. When dry, you may wish to add a light touch of hair spray, nonlacquer type.

For good-looking control, Wig Spray Patene is recommended. Your wig set will easily outlast your own natural hair set, since wig hair isn't slept on and has no natural oils to flatten or soil it. To help retain the good looks of your wig, avoid wearing it in rain, strong winds, or bright sunlight. Wig-wearing at home has its advantages.

The quality of today's synthetics easily rivals that of human-hair wigs both in looks and ease of care. Care of synthetics differs only slightly from the real thing. Often synthetics come with their own built-in set, and while this may make restyling next to impossible, it also means easier care, no need to spray, fewer washings, no limp, loose, or frizzy look, even in the worst of weather. Fibers such as Dynel can be washed, styled, packed, and restyled almost effortlessly. Synthetic hairpieces come clean with water and a little detergent. Cold-water Woolite is often recommended. Check the directions which come with the hairpiece. If the fake is either a synthetic fall or a switch, place it in a nylon net bag before you clean or wash it. To dry, hang it full-length on a hanger over a towel and let it drip dry. For synthetic wigs and wiglets, place on a wig block and let dry at room temeprature. Avoid frizzing and melting by never placing your synthetic wig under a hot dryer. It's just that simple.

19.
Hairpieces for Men, Hair Weaving, Transplants

"The hair is real, it's the head that's fake," said a well-known Hollywood actor on being asked if he wore a toupee.

The statement generally typifies the attitude of a serious male wig wearer. Those men who are concerned enough to want a hairpiece in order to improve their image, often go to extremes to keep the real truth a secret. So good are today's hairpieces for men that a girl might never know. Men's hairpieces can be slept in, showered in, and can even survive the most vigorous swim sessions. More men than a girl can possibly suspect are suddenly making it by faking it; over a million men now sport newly acquired hair.

It used to be that a man wearing a hairpiece to cover his barren head was considered a prime target for a joke. Today's laughs are for the uninformed. Credit for better hairpieces for men goes to the movie and television producers who, in an attempt to maintain the youthful looks of male stars, prompted wig manufacturers to turn out more natural-looking pieces. In an age of hair consciousness where youth spells success, show

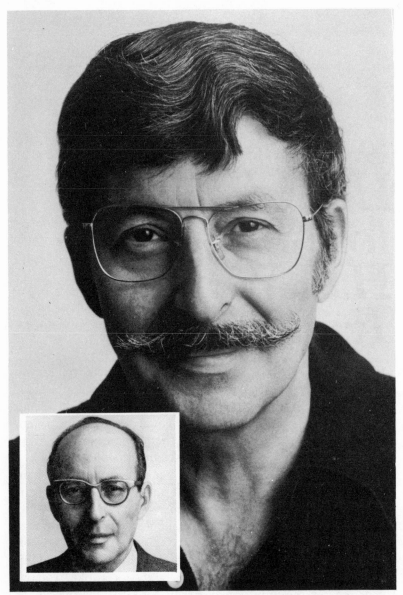

At Penthouse for Men, N.Y.C., secure in the knowledge that even experts have trouble spotting them, more and more men are taking advantage of a "second head of hair."

biz personalities, businessmen, professional leaders, salesmen, and even the fellow next-door are easy candidates for hairpieces. Those with the yen to look younger, or more romantic, or more disitnguished, or more mysterious, or more anything are turning to men's hairpieces.

Veterans of Vietnam, too, are discovering wigs as a cover-up for temporary baldness or scarring from a scalp wound. A temporary wig often gives the boost necessary for total recovery. The United States government has authorized the Veteran's Bureau to issue wigs to veterans who are eligible to receive medical care and treatment for hair loss. For veterans and nonvets alike, if a doctor prescribes a wig, it can be shown as an income-tax deduction. That's progress! Neither Hannibal, who wore a wig while crossing the Alps nor Julius Ceasar, who used a laurel wreath to crown his shiny head, ever secured such fringe benefits.

Present estimates indicate that 75 percent of the male population over forty show some sign of baldness. In some instances, hair loss is temporary and reversible. Infections with high fever accompanying, hormonal imbalance, drugs, or even severe emotional strain can be the cause of sudden loss of hair. Under any of these circumstances, it is possible to restore hair provided proper medical help is sought in time. Gradual hair loss, which starts with a receding hairline, merely indicates male-pattern baldness for which science still seeks a cure. Our present mode of remedy is that of cosmetic correction through hair styling or, in more severe cases, reverting to hair pieces, hair weaving, or hair transplants. The least painful of the correctives is a hairpiece and, while it may not be a permanent remedy, it is likely to be less costly and less time-consuming. Secure in the knowledge that even experts have trouble spotting them, more and more men are taking advantage of today's improved male cover-ups.

Cover-ups vary in size from the total Beatle wig to the toupee which covers only the wide-open spaces on top and blends in with remaining side and back fringes, to hairpieces which cover a small area, usually worn up front to cover a receding hairlines.

Then there are special "problem pieces" used to cover difficult empty or thinning spots.

Rather than resorting to a full wig, most men prefer to use a well-styled hairpiece to fill in a receding hairlines or a bald spot. Now there's a new way to make sure the piece stays put surgically. A stitch here, a stitch there, strategically placed, affix the hairpiece to the head on a semi permanent basis. It is best to discuss the process with your doctor as the risk of infection though minimal, exists. The cost of a man's hairpiece varies according to the size area that needs covering and color blending requirements.

A man doesn't have to be a bigwig to own a wig. He doesn't even have to live in or near a big city. The Sears and Roebuck Company now makes wigs available on a mail-order basis. The catalog offers hairpieces in a variety of styles for men and includes a tape measure, a paper pattern for indicating head size and shape, an envelope for samples of the hair to be matched, and instructions for measuring. So far, the mail-order business seems to be paying off handsomely for all concerned.

What price glory? For a man whose hair is receding on one side of his forehead, hairpieces are available for about $55. If both sides present a problem, the price usually goes up to $135. When a bald area measures about five-by-seven inches, the cost runs close to $300, and if a "problem piece" is required the price can grow as high as $1,000.

The best male wigs, toupees, and hairpieces are made from undyed, untreated hair, usually imported from Europe. Although oriental hair is cheaper, it doesn't match Western hair in texture. To achieve realistic results, shades of commercial European hair are painstakingly color-matched to the customer's own hair. (Dyeing is a dead give-away.) For a perfect fit, the base is hand-sewn. Since men wear hairpieces consistently, a second hairpiece is usually needed so one can be cleaned while the other one is being worn. Often men own several pieces in alternating styles and lengths to simulate hair growth. Provided a toupee or hairpiece is cleaned at least once a month, it should last up to three years.

Goatees, sideburns, and mustaches are presently growing in demand. These new additions are usually reserved for weekend use. Purchase price depends on style; a man can get a mustache for as little as $7.95 in a choice of traditional, drooping, or contintental styles; sideburns sell for $12.95; beards for $19.95. In less than one-half hour a fellow can transform himself into a Bond Street gentleman, a wigged-out Edwardian, or a continental playboy; all it takes is the right equipment and some theatrical spirit gum.

Sideburns, beards, and mustaches are easy to apply and are fun variety pieces. Knowing there is little likelihood of running into old girl friends, GIs often take advantage of these trick pieces to perk up weekend leaves.

Although most men are generally discreet about any form of wig wear, those who sport accessory hairpieces are not at all self-conscious. After all, they argue, if a girl can wear false eyelashes why can't a guy wear false sideburns or a goatee if he's in the mood and the time is right?

The men have a point. In principle, they're only catching on to what females have been doing for a long time. The truth is, if a man can gain greater assurance, more joy, a better job, and improve his love life by merely resorting to a hairpiece he would be foolish to turn down such possibilities.

Hair Weaving

Hair weaving is a relatively new means of camouflage. Some consider this home-grown/hand-sewn combination to be the next best thing to growing God-given hair. The majority of hair-weaving enthusiasts are men. (Most women remain content to pop on a wig or wiglet to conceal their woes.) Beauticians, however, cater to both sexes. For that matter, black beauticians have for a good number of years utilized the technique to achieve a long-straight look for patrons desiring straight hair without resorting to harsh, bad-smelling hair products. Hair weaving is available to all regardless of sex or race. As a result, many new heads are turning to hair weaving as a means of salvation.

The only prerequisite for hair weaving is that the candidate have a sufficient number of natural hairs on the head with which to work. Thinning hair, a receding hairline, and a bald spot are all problems which can be overcome through hair weaving. A totally bald head does not lend itself to this technique.

In a hair-weave process, an individual's own hair is utilized together with nylon threads which are interwoven with the natural hair to form a meshlike base close to the scalp wherever hair is thin or barren. Hanks of matching hair are then sewn into the base. Between the newly hand-sewn hair and the original home-grown, an expert can raise a hardy crop of healthy looking hair.

Unlike most toupees, since the hair is not glued or taped, it doesn't ever come off, unless requested. Besides the fact that the wearer can sleep, shower, swim or participate in any other sport he chooses without fear of exposure, there are strong psychological advantages. Hair-weaving enthusiasts grow to consider their new hair to be a real part of themselves, just as fingernails and teeth are, Actually, the relationship between hair weaving and a hairpiece is similar to a capped tooth versus removable bridgework.

Accomplishing the hair-weave process takes three to four hours. The minimum cost usually runs $375; but cost does not stop there. Since honest-to-goodness hair continues to grow, the base and hank of hairs sewn to it gradually move out as real hair gets longer. This means that adjustments are necessary every two or three months for which the service fee can be as much as $50.

Because there are no standards for licensing, and although they are likely to be few and far between, problems can arise. Dr. Hillard H. Pearlstein, a member of the Orentreich Medical Group in New York City, on examining thirty hair-woven scalps, found that in cases where serious dandruff existed the condition worsened under the woven base and that the base itself contributed to exacerbating an unclean scalp condition. Subsequent to his initial finding, Dr. Pearlstein later discovered one hair-weave client with traction alopecia, a form of baldness caused by scalp tension. This time it wasn't a too tightly pulled ponytail which was at fault but rather the woven mesh base which was too tightly anchored to the real hair and which, in turn, caused natural hairs to be literally pulled out by their roots.

In this particular case, the hair loss was reversible because the situation could be corrected in time. Any discomfort of a hair-woven scalp should be reported and remedied immediately. If hair is continually pulled out by the roots over an extended period of time, eventually it will not be able to grow back.

Although the case discussed appears to be rather exceptional, a word of caution is in order regarding the selection of a hair weave expert. If you want to get it sewn up right, check it out first.

Transplants

Transplants are the newest form of cosmetic correction making headline news. Thousands of male heads, some of them celebrated, have already flipped their wigs in favor of hair transplants. This new surgical technique has produced mighty impressive results in resodding barren scalps.

The process is relatively simple. By means of, essentially, a skin-graft technique, hair is transplanted from lush crops to areas which are sparse or barren. Although the subject at hand is obviously not gardening, for the sake of simplification, we may liken hair to grass. In the case of hair transplants, the grass is definitely not greener in anyone else's backyard. For that matter, the only grass that can be used for refurbishing is that which already exists within your own topsoil. This means there must be donor land from which to draw.

As it happens, male-pattern baldness offers just such an area. On the male head, hair recedes slowly, creeping back until, in the final stage, all that remains is a U-shaped fringe of hair just ample enough for transplant purposes. To be successful, transplanting should be carried out only after the final pattern of baldness has been established. Transplanting done too early may force new growth to fall by the wayside during the course of continued balding.

Resodding sessions are becoming an almost commonplace happening in medical offices throughout the country. The individuals most responsible for the techniques used by both dermatologists and plastic surgeons are such doctors as Ayers, Lubowe, Blau, Berger, Orentreich, Feit, and Vallis; dedicated men from coast to coast who have developed a hair-redistribution system based on a skin-graft technique entailing use of local anesthesia, usually Novocaine. The combined efforts of these men have made possible the successful removal of small grafts of hair—(technically named plugs)—from the side and back areas of the head where hair tends to be more plentiful, and transplant the very same plugs to barren areas on the top of the head where hair is needed most. Patches are able to remain in their new location due to clotting. Although stitches are not absolutely necessary, some doctors prefer to close the donor areas through painless suturing. The successful transplant of grassylike patches has been a big help in closing the generation gap, principally for men. It is no wonder that other professionals and their patients joyously take off their hats in salute to the celebrated works of these men.

Despite the many excellent results, plug transplants are not yet all a bed of roses. There are several thorns. Costs run high, doctor vists are many, and results are often slow and painstaking. On the average, each graft contains ten to fifteen hairs. An average of one hundred grafts are needed to resod a well-receded hairline; two hundred grafts or more are needed for severe balding. Normally, twenty to fifty grafts can be accomplished at sessions spaced at least a week apart. Depending upon the severity of balding, numerous visits are needed over the course of several months for complete cover-up. It

Hair Tranplants (Plug Type)

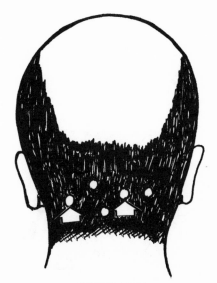

DONOR AREA

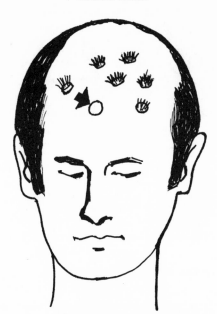

RECIPIENT AREA

Raising of Bilobe Hair Flaps and Rotating Them to Recreate Frontal Hairline

SURGICAL STEPS   PHYSICAL RESULTS

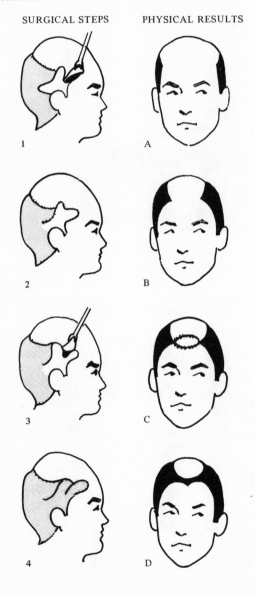

Galeaplasty (A Surgical Technique to Stop Further Hair Loss and Promote Better Growth)

A, B, C and D indicate the surgical steps taken to stimulate the vascular and lymphatic bed and the mobilization of the under-surface of the galea to bring about improved hair growth and to diminish further loss.

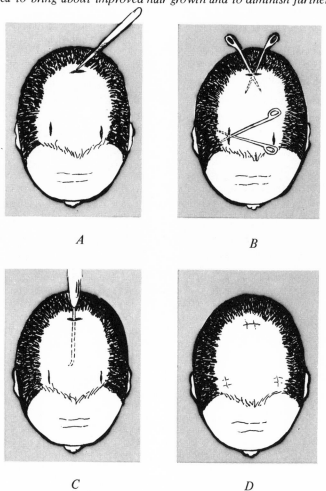

A

B

C

D

takes approximately three months for the new hairs, which initially have a cornstalk appearance, to become firmly embedded and to show all the normal signs of life and growth. Patches may be in the form of plugs, strips, or flaps, depending on the doctor's technique. Scars blend with their surroundings after a few months. If patches are sparse and thin to begin with, transplants, too, will be skimpy.

What price glamour? With costs ranging from $5 to $25 per plug, the total capital for resodding can run anywhere between $500 and $3000.

These conditions (among others) prompted Dr. Louis J. Feit, director of plastic surgery at New York Polyclinic Medical School and Hospital, to search along similar paths for a more efficient means of attacking the problem, and to seek a method to avoid further hair loss, and also to improve the chances of transplant results. His work led him to develop a surgical technique which he calls galeaplasty. Where medical or dermatological care have failed, galeaplasty is used to change the nutritional base of the bald area, to encourage hair growth, and to stop further hair loss. The term *galeaplasty* is used since the central bald area is referred to as the region of *galea aponeurotica*. Galeaplasty is akin to replowing topsoil as a means to stimulate growth of lusher crops. Dr. Feit accomplishes this by changing the vascular and lymphatic beds, and mobilizing the undersurface of the galea. Whether natural or transplanted, hair growth is stimulated by this method.

In the area of transplants, Dr. Feit observed that the removal of ten to fifteen hairs in a small button clump ultimately left a sparse donor area and created honeycomb scarring in some cases in the recipient area. Too many hairs taken from a single donor area might, in fact, redistribute baldness rather than successfully cover up barren territory. As a result, Dr. Feit developed a further technique called the bilobe flap, used chiefly to restore the frontal hairline in almost one clip. According to the doctor, "Once the patient has a natural-looking front, he is generally satisfied. If he is concerned about the back area he may elect to intensify this area with sod implants, patches, or strips, or, if content with the frontal line, may simply wear a small, comfortably fitting hairpiece."

Dr. Feit's technique is to take a flap containing 1000 to 2000 hairs from each side of the head; however, rather than removing a graft, he creates a flap of hair and rotates it toward the frontal hairline to recreate the original hairline. Actually, the hair-bearing skin is donated from the neck where it is very mobile and pushed forward; no replacement graft is required. Since the base and the bilobe flap carry the main trunk of the superficial temporal artery, the transplanted area becomes revitalized with both hair and health. Any scalp tensions which might have existed in the previously barren area are eliminated because of improved circulatory conditions in that area. Patch grafts are used to close up the center openings on top. So long as the flaps are healthy in their original location, they will continue to grow with equal health in their new location. Surgical and cosmetic results based upon Dr. Feit's technique of using flaps rather than many small patches have been excellent.

In cases where hair transplants do not become firmly embedded and thus are not successful, failure can, in certain instances, attributed by some physicians directly to the patient's lack of adequate nutrition. A diet consisting of an overabundance of carbohydrates and insufficient protein intake, coupled with smoking, are two strikes against transplant success. Vitamins are important in connection with supplying the energy to bring about changes.

In view of the greater problems which men must confront, they will undoubtedly remain the best candidates for hair transplants. By comparison, women don't seem to show a plugged nickel's worth of interest in the whole affair despite the fact that Dr. Orentreich recommends hair transplants when female baldness is of the male-pattern type.

It should be remembered that hair transplants are a relatively new form of treatment and have only been in commercial use for less than a decade. Further study, research, and exploration may result in new and better forms of cover-up techniques. Transplants are an important step in this direction.

20.
Evaluating Commercial Hair Systems

A prominent dermatologist estimates that exclusive of physicians' fees and prescription costs men spend $7 billion a year on hair. No one knows for sure what amount is actually expended fruitlessly on systems, services and useless products.

"New hair in ten weeks. . . ." "Permanent hair in two hours!" "A full head of hair in three to four hours. . . ." Companies X, Y, and Z all make hair-raising promises, but the question is, do they really pay off?

As with horse racing and other forms of gambling, hair systems don't always work out profitably. Certain approaches or systems may be helpful to certain individuals. At least an acute interest in any one of the so-called systems is indicative of an awareness of a particular problem. Most systems are intended for men, although a few attempt to include women in their fold as well. Some of the systems guaranteeing more hair are well-meaning operations, others are purely commercial endeavors. Some are filled with half-truths, and others merely distortions of the truth. Some systems will work on the heads of some people; others will work for other people; some will never work at all. Success is dependent on the person and his or her problem, as well as on the so-called cure. If you hope to make substantial headway, keep in mind that for serious hair problems, your own family doctor or dermatologist is the very best source of advice. Nevertheless, many persist in seeking help through other sources. As long as you know what is possible and what is not, judging the merits of any system of approach is greatly simplified.

Magazines and certain big-city dailies offer more advertising to acquire hair than you can possibly shake your missing locks at. Often, regardless of whether they are based on wig wear, hair weaving, or programs for stimulating hair growth, the before-and-after results appear most impressive. Openings such as those that follow are typical. Before signing your name on any contractual agreement or on your check, be sure to look into the offer carefully. Don't be browbeaten into any program that factually cannot work for you. Although reading helps to keep you aware, in the case of unvarnished advertising, the message very often is simply to beware.

Energize your scalp to help produce thicker hair. . . .

We will start new hair growth within ten weeks or your money back. . . .

Balding—hair's a way to end it. Regain some of your youthful appearance—our natural method hairweave.

Thumbs down on baldness. If you're not satisfied within 30 days, the money you have paid for treatment will be refunded. You're the sole judge.

Balding—try minimax silicon hairpiece and see how much younger and vital you can be.

Medical breakthrough gives permanent hair in just 2 hours. Not a toupee, transplant, hairweave or wig. . . .

Loss of hair through neglect. For the first time a 4-way home treatment. Here's your guarantee. Examine your hair before and after 30 days. Dandruff should be eliminated, your scalp relieved, hair cleaner, thicker, more alive. If you don't see a thrilling improvement, your money will be refunded.

A dream yesterday, a reality today. Permanent hair without weaving or transplants.

If you're going to advance upon the receding hairline and be successful, you make sure to treat only those on whom the treatment will work. After seven to ten treatments you see and judge the results. Improvements have resulted in every instance.

As an added headline, there is this final addition: to distinguish between fact and fiction means keeping up-to-date with the latest developments. As research continues in an attempt to pinpoint the causes and cures for hair loss, new theories and techniques continue to arise while older theories are either reconfirmed or discarded. Through trial and error, a multitude of so-called systems for hair improvement flash on the scene in addition to those currently in operation. Any evaluation of publicly advertised systems of hair improvement must be made within a framework of ever-expanding factual knowledge. If this were not so, medicine men might still be hawking the wonders of bear's oil for growing hair.

The last word on the subject of systems is—stay on top of all new discoveries. Read the literature, review the facts and be your own judge.

21.
Hair –
Past, Present and Future

Not since the days of Samson and Delilah has hair played such havoc in the lives of men. The real roots of the hirsute scene, however, date back to the earliest days of mankind; Stone Age graffiti reveal that in those lusty days a well-bred caveman selected the woman of his choice by grabbing her up by the roots of her hair.

From recorded annals we learn that Thutmos III, a bigwig of ancient Egypt, added homelike touches to his tomb by burying his treasures with him, including no less than three shoulder-length wigs belonging to his wives, Princesses Menwi, Merti, and Menhet, doubtlessly the most wigged-out trio of 1450 B.C.

Throughout the ages, women have been making history by using their heads to advantage. Cleopatra's private secret may well have been her coal-tar henna rinses. How far would Lady Godiva have ridden had it not been for her flowing locks? A towering three-foot-tall coiffure perhaps gave Marie Antoinette her biggest boost. On the other hand, Mary Queen of Scots, with only a scanty head of hair, ended her days by wearing a wig to her own execution.

Queen Victoria is known to have been a collector of hair tropies. Her most valued possesssions were a brooch containing a lock of her mother's hair and a bracelet with a secret compartment in which she carried a lock of Prince Albert's hair. Hair collecting gained added momentum in the eighteenth century when Frenchmen began dangling pocket watches from chains of woven human hair, usually the hair of a departed loved one. Hair collecting at last took on commercial proportions during Victorian days. A quote from an enterprising ad of the times reads: "Hair is at once the most delicate and lasting material and survives us like love. It is so light, so gentle, so escaping from the idea of death, that with a lock of hair belonging to a child or friend, we may almost look up to heaven and compare notes with angelic nature—may almost say 'I have a piece of thee here, not unworthy of thy being now.' " Underlying such attitudes is the belief that treasured locks symbolize a total being.

Japanese culture has clung to a variation of this belief for years. For many centuries the royal hair of the Mikado could be cut only when he slept as it was presumed that only at that time did his soul safely flee his body. Hair cutting during waking hours was deemed ill-timed and detrimental to the Mikado's mental and physical powers.

Today, a similar theory survives on the tiny Dutch island of Amboyna. According to islanders, a man's soul and strength are bound up with his hair. Not so surprising, then, that justice in Amboyna often triumphs as the island's court barber waves a shiny pair of scissors before the accused. Where physical torture fails, the threat of the shears succeeds in obtaining the hair-raising truth in Amboyna. The psychological value of hair cannot be underestimated.

In our culture, hair power surpasses flower power, as well as nearly every other power. Hair is where the action is. To be part of the swinging discotheque crowd, GIs in Paris and Frankfurt spend $15 to $30 for weekend wig rentals. In London, GIs make the scene by renting phony mustaches at a cost of $4 to

$10 per weekend. Check out your TV set—is that cool, hip musician swinging his own luxuruous locks? Is that smiling emcee scratching his own head of hair? Does he or doesn't he? Only his hairdresser knows for sure.

People of all ages are taking a second look in the mirror and those who want to get ahead are emphasizing their hair in order to advance their careers. The wigged-out include not only matrons, business and professional women, models, actresses, and grandmothers, but now actors, GIs, salesmen, and businessmen are also wigging ahead to boost their morale and their careers.

Today, liberation for all mankind lies just around the bend, when it will no longer be possible to label who or what a person is by his style of dress or by the cut of his hair. Whether it's curly, frizzy, snaggy, shaggy, ratty, shining, gleaming, streaming, knotted, twisted, beaded, powdered, flowered, bangled, tangled or spangled. . . . "Show it, long as God can grow it." "HAIR!"

Looking ahead, where hair is concerned, the future gleams with an out-of-sight new sparkle. One of the most sophisticated hair happenings today is the recent use of the Optico Screen Microscope. By means of this innovation a sample hair strand is projected on microtelevision for thorough, instant analysis and diagnosis. According to the reassuring words of Dr. Norman Orentreich, "As new facts are uncovered, the day of medical control of all aspects of hair growth comes closer and closer." Scientific study and research offer many promising new advances for the years to come.

Hair authority Leslie Blanchard predicts an amazing possibility. It may not be too long before you'll be able to sip a magic potion or swallow a pill and *zap*— overnight, your natural hair color will be transformed into just the shade you choose, even the most subtle blond tones you've ever imagined.

Microphotography offers yet another possibility. With proper development, the day may come when beauty counters everywhere will feature microphotography to view single strands of hair as a means of diagnosing hair problems while a transistorized computer feeds back answers to hair concerns and prescribes solutions instantly.

Hypnosis, too, offers another unexplored powerhouse of potential. Through developments in both autosuggestion and hypnosis, a subject might simply be told to reverse the process of balding to whatever state he or she desires. The underlying inference is that when the mind is in the right place, under hypnosis, the body will automatically understand what it needs to restore or create hair growth. The other inference is that the substances to make it happen are available within the body and, in fact, are at the subject's own command. Needless to say, success of autosuggestion as a means of correcting hair ills depends to a major extent on greater exploration, but in it may well lie the answers to many age-old problems.

When William Shakespeare wrote, "Time himself is bald and therefore to the world's end will have bald followers," he obviously knew of what he wrote. The same timeless vibrations which inspired Shakespeare are equally compelling forces for today's scientists and astrologers engrossed in the study of the universal dynamics governing all life forms, including that of hair. New knowledge of electrical impulses and magnetics within the universe may soon lead to personalized hair horoscopes charting the exact day, hour, and precise moment for hair's good growth, motion, magnetic thickening, development of strenght, dynamic regeneration, or propensive penetration, which simply means the best time to get a haircut.

Everything seems to be looking up. If the promises of the politicians materialize, soon we'll be able to hold our heads high without a worry or care concerning pollution, soot, or smog. It is, of course, conceivable that the future holds new problems in store, but, if we get together now, perhaps we will not have to contend with such eventual problems as radiation or its effects on health or hair.

Until future happenings become a reality, practice the art of living the realities of now. Let your hair down, investigate, experiment, discover the fun of synthetics, take advantage of all the new products on the market, give your hair all the love and care you can. The hair care you give today is your door opener to facing the future more beautifully—tomorrow.

Index